Sheela Rao

16/9/05

The Effective Management of
Upper Gastrointestinal Malignancies

May 2005.

Dear Sheela,

I deal reading for your next vacation.

David.

Thanks for all your help.

Titles of related interest in the UK Key Advances in Clinical Practice Series

SOLID TUMOURS

The Effective Management of Breast Cancer, 1st and 2nd edns
The Effective Management of Colorectal Cancer, 1st, 2nd, 3rd and 4th edns
The Effective Management of Lung Cancer, 1st, 2nd and 3rd edns
The Effective Management of Malignant Melanoma
The Effective Management of Ovarian Cancer, 1st, 2nd and 3rd edns
The Effective Management of Prostatic Cancer
The Effective Management of Renal Cell Carcinoma
The Effective Management of Urological Cancer

HAEMATOLOGICAL MALIGNANCIES

The Effective Management of Non-Hodgkin's Lymphoma, 1st and 2nd edns
The Effective Prevention and Management of Systemic Fungal Infection in Haematological
Malignancy, 1st and 2nd edns
The Effective Management of Common Complications of Induction Chemotherapy in
Haematological Malignancy
The Effective Management of Chronic Lymphocytic Leukaemia

SYMPTOM CONTROL

The Effective Management of Cancer Pain, 1st and 2nd edns
The Effective Prevention and Control of Symptoms in Cancer
The Effective Prevention and Management of Post-Operative Nausea
& Vomiting, 1st and 2nd edns

HEALTH POLICY

NICE, CHI and the NHS Reforms: Enabling excellence or imposing control?
Clinical Governance and the NHS Reforms: Enabling excellence or imposing control?
Managed Care Networks: Principles and practice

The Effective Management of Upper Gastrointestinal Malignancies

Edited by

David Cunningham MD FRCP
Consultant Medical Oncologist & Head, GI and Lymphoma Units,
The Royal Marsden Hospital, London and Surrey, UK

Janusz Jankowski MD PhD FRCP
Professor of Gastroenterology and Medicine & Director,
Digestive Diseases Centre, Department of Medicine and Oncology,
University of Leicester, UK

Andrew Miles MSc MPhil PhD
Professor of Public Health Sciences,
Editor-in-Chief, Journal of Evaluation in Clinical Practice,
Barts and The London,
Queen Mary's School of Medicine and Dentistry, University of London, UK

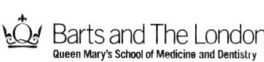

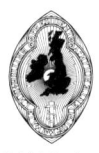

British Society
for
Gastroenterology

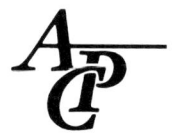

Association of
Cancer
Physicians

The Royal College
of
Radiologists

AESCULAPIUS MEDICAL PRESS
LONDON SAN FRANCISCO SYDNEY

Published by

Aesculapius Medical Press (London, San Francisco, Sydney)
PO Box LB48, London EC1A 1LB, UK

British Library Cataloguing in Publication Data
A CIP catalogue record for this book is available from the British Library

ISBN: 1 903044 45 6

While the advice and information in this book are believed to be true and accurate at the
time of going to press, neither the authors nor the publishers nor the sponsoring institutions
can accept any legal responsibility or liability for errors or omissions that may be made.
In particular (but without limiting the generality of the preceding disclaimer) every effort
has been made to check drug usages; however, it is possible that errors have been missed.
Furthermore, dosage schedules are constantly being revised and new side effects recognised.
For these reasons, the reader is strongly urged to consult the drug companies' printed
instructions before administering any of the drugs recommended in this book.

Further copies of this volume are available from:

Claudio Melchiorri
Aesculapius Medical Press
PO Box LB48, Mount Pleasant Mail Centre, Farringdon Road, London EC1A 1LB, UK

Fax: 020 8525 8661
Email: claudio@keyadvances4.demon.co.uk

Copy edited by The Clyvedon Press Ltd, Cardiff, UK

Typeset, printed and bound in Britain
Peter Powell Origination & Print Limited

Contents

Contributors

William Allum FRCS, Consultant Upper GI Surgeon, The Royal Marsden Hospital, London and Surrey & National Clinical Lead for Upper GI Cancer Services Improvement Programme

Anne C. Armstrong MB ChB MRCP, Specialist Registrar in Medical Oncology, Department of Medical Oncology, Christie Hospital NHS Trust, Manchester, UK

Stephen Attwood BA (Mod) MCh FRCS FRCSI (Gen), Consultant Surgeon, North Tyneside General Hospital, Tyneside

Hugh Barr ChM MD FRCS FRCSE ILTM, Professor and Consultant Upper GI Surgeon, Gloucester Royal Hospital, Gloucester, UK

Carlos Caldas MD FACP FRCP, Senior Investigator, Cancer Genomics Programme and Honorary Consultant Medical Oncologist, Hutchison-MRC Research Centre, Addenbrooke's Hospital and University of Cambridge, UK

Ian Chau MBBS MRCP, Clinical Research Fellow, Department of Medicine and Gastrointestinal Unit, Royal Marsden Hospital, Sutton, Surrey, UK

Adrian Crellin FRCP FRCR, Consultant Clinical Oncologist, Leeds Cancer Centre, UK

David Cunningham MD FRCP, Consultant Medical Oncologist, Head of Department of Medicine and Gastrointestinal Unit, Royal Marsden Hospital, Sutton, Surrey, UK

James Dickson MBBS, Clinical Research Fellow, Department of Medicine and Gastrointestinal Unit, Royal Marsden Hospital, Sutton, Surrey, UK

Clare Donnellan MBBS BSc MRCP, Research Registrar in Gastroenterology, Leeds General Infirmary, UK

Simon Everett MBChB MRCP MD, Consultant in Gastroenterology, Leeds General Infirmary, UK

David Forman BA PhD FFPHM, Professor of Cancer Epidemiology, University of Leeds, UK

Rebecca C. Fitzgerald MA MD MRCP, MRC Group Leader and Honorary Specialist Registrar in Gastroenterology, Hutchison-MRC Research Centre, Addenbrooke's Hospital and University of Cambridge, UK

Daniel Hochhauser DPhil FRCP, Kathleen-Ferrier Reader in Medical Oncology, The Royal Free and University College Medical School, London, UK

Martin Hogg MA BMBS FRCR, Specialist Registrar, Christie Hospital NHS Trust, Manchester, UK

Janusz A. Jankowski MD PhD FRCP, Professor of Gastroenterology and Medicine, Departments of Medicine and Oncology, University of Leicester, UK

Vincent S. Khoo MBBS FRACR MD, Senior Lecturer in Clinical Oncology, Christie Hospital NHS Trust, Manchester, UK

Paul Moayyedi BSc MB ChB MPH PhD FRCP, Professor of Gastroenterology, McMaster University, Hamilton, Canada

Satvinder S. Mudan BSc MB BS MD FRCS, Consultant in Surgical Oncology, The Royal Marsden Hospital, London and Surrey, UK

Marianne C. Nicolson MD BSc FRCP, Consultant Medical Oncologist, Aberdeen Royal Infirmary and Department of Medicine and Therapeutics, University of Aberdeen, Aberdeen, UK

Russell D. Petty MB MRCP, Department of Oncology, Aberdeen Royal Infirmary and Department of Medicine and Therapeutics, University of Aberdeen, Aberdeen, UK

Sheela Rao MBBS MRCP, Clinical Research Fellow, Department of Medicine and Gastrointestinal Unit, Royal Marsden Hospital, Sutton, Surrey, UK

Mark P. Saunders MBBS MRCP FRCR PhD, Consultant Clinical Oncologist and Honorary Clinical Lecturer, Christie Hospital NHS Trust and Paterson Institute, Manchester, UK

Nicholas C. Turner MA MRCP, Specialist Registrar in Medical Oncology, Middlesex Hospital, London, UK

Juan W. Valle MB ChB MRCP MSc, Senior Lecturer and Honorary Consultant, Department of Medical Oncology, Christie Hospital NHS Trust, Manchester, UK

Peter Watson BSc MD FRCP FRCPI, Senior Lecturer in Medicine, Queens University, Belfast & Consultant Gastroenterologist, Belfast Victoria Hospital, Belfast

Ian M. Welch BSc MB ChB PhD FRCS, Consultant Oesophago-Gastric Surgeon, Christie Hospital NHS Trust, Manchester, UK

Chris Williams PhD, Cochrane Cancer Network, Institute of Health Sciences, Oxford, UK

Preface

Each year, upper gastrointestinal cancers cause nearly 1 million deaths. Epidemiologically, they are characterised by enormous variability according to geographical location, gender and ethnic group and in recent decades there have been profound changes in their incidence. Distal gastric cancer, for example, is reducing whereas the incidence of oesophageal and gastric cardia adenocarcinomas is, on the contrary, rising. It is becoming increasingly apparent that definitive environmental factors are of direct significance to the aetiology and development of upper gastrointestinal malignancies. Indeed, as Donnellan, Forman and Everett point out in the opening chapter of this volume, the pathogenesis of oesophageal squamous cell cancer is closely associated with tobacco smoking and, to a lesser extent, exposure to alcohol. In terms of distal gastric cancer, the most powerful risk factor has been identified as infection with *Helicobacter pylori* and the reducing incidence of this cancer is probably due to the declining frequency of prolonged infection. It is noteworthy, as the authors discuss, that recent data have shown that some individuals with specific polymorphisms of genes encoding pro-inflammatory and anti-inflammatory cytokines, two of which (IL-1 and TNF-alpha) are also potent acid inhibitors, are predisposed to develop corpus-predominant gastritis, gastric atrophy and gastric cancer as a result of *H. pylori* infection. A comparison, for example, of Japanese individuals who are typically at high risk of gastric cancer with English subjects who are typically at low risk of the disease, has shown accelerated atrophy and corpus gastritis in response to *H. pylori* infection, independent of strain type, in Japanese individuals. The debate as to whether *H. pylori* protects against GORD and junctional cancers remains, on the other hand, essentially unresolved and the greatest protective effect of *H. pylori* appears to be in those people susceptible to corpus predominant gastritis and thus any protective effect of *H. pylori* against junctional cancers will mainly in those most at risk of distal gastric cancer. These data, as Donnellan and colleagues conclude, confirm that upper gastrointestinal malignancies develop as a result of complicated interactions between environmental factors and genetic predisposition.

It is to a specific consideration of the molecular and clinical genetics of upper gastrointestinal malignancies that Fitzgerald and Caldas turn in Chapter Two. As these authors discuss, a small percentage of oesophago-gastric cancers occur as a result of clearly identified cancer predisposition syndromes and the potential to identify affected asymptomatic individuals has clear and far reaching consequences for patient management, particularly in relation to the utility of appropriately designed surveillance strategies and the use of prophylactic surgery. An example employed by the authors is the identification of E-cadherin mutations in hereditary diffuse gastric cancer. Here, as well as the heritable effect of high-penetrance genes, there are also low-penetrance genes which may contribute to common sporadic cancers and these observations are of direct and clear importance to a large proportion of the population. These low penetrance genes are harder to identify and any carcinogenesis will almost certainly be influenced by exposure to environmental triggers, a good example being the contribution of interleukin-1 polymorphisms in determining the risk for the development of gastric cancer in *H.pylori* infected individuals. Within upper gastrointestinal tissues, the sequence of somatic mutations has also been studied with the aim of identifying clinically relevant bio-markers. But as Fitzgerald and Caldas point out, it is increasingly recognised that there are a large number of target genes involved which do not necessarily follow an obligate linear sequence and the final common pathway for these somatic mutations is uncontrolled cell proliferation. In the premalignant condition Barrett's oesophagus, there is evidence that a novel proliferation marker called minichromosome maintenance protein, may have the potential to predict patients at risk for cancer development. Furthermore, with the advent of gene expression profiling analysis of the global gene expression profile of these cancers, and their precursors, clinical advances are likely to be made in terms of predicting cancer risk and response to treatment.

The incidence of oesophageal adenocarcinomas is increasing in the Western world as Donnellan and associates documented in Chapter One, but the poor prognosis of the disease is due principally to the characteristic late presentation of the patient with definitive symptoms and the accompanying late stage of disease. In Chapter Three, which closes Part One of this volume, Jankowski and his co-authors provide an overview of current thinking on the benefits of intervention and surveillance strategies for Barrett's oesophagus. The conversion rate for Barrett's metaplasia is higher in the UK than anywhere else and while attempts to intervene at an earlier stage of tumour progression have not been shown to be cost-effective, lesions identified during surveillance programs undoubtedly have a better prognosis. Consequently, there has been renewed interest in the development and use of strategies that may prevent the precursor lesion Barrett's oesophagus and of clear importance to this particular field of enquiry is our significantly improved understanding of the gene-environmental interactions necessary for the clonal expansion, and hence propagation, of metaplastic premalignant lesions. It is clear, as Jankowski et al discuss, that three mechanisms – including inheritance of germ-line mutations, sporadic mutagenesis and local epigenetic alterations – promote cancer progression. In Barrett's oesophagus, there have been no inherited genetic mutations identified to date and it therefore appears likely that locally produced cytokines and bile and acid in the refluxate create a microenvironment that sets the scene for metaplastic transformation of the oesophageal epithelium. It is precisely the conceptual understanding of the pathogenesis of this condition, as well as chronic mucosal inflammation elsewhere such as the stomach and colon, that is likely to lead to improved therapeutic intervention. Specifically, inhibition of chronic mucosal inflammation and of the activation of dietary carcinogens are considered by the authors to represent cheap and effective interventions as part of a logical and viable approach to the effective management of patients who have been identified as at clear risk.

Although the late stage of disease at presentation continues to represent a major factor in determining clinical outcome from therapy, it is nevertheless true to recognise that earlier diagnosis of upper gastrointestinal malignancy is occurring as the result of the increased availability of open access endoscopy and surveillance programmes for patients with Barrett's oesophagus. Distinction between squamous cell carcinoma and adenocarcinoma of the oesophagus is important as it affects patient management in many units. A number of rarer malignancies arise in the oesophagus and their diagnosis also frequently alters management. The assessment of dysplasia in both the oesophagus and the stomach may be difficult and repeat biopsies required. A second expert pathological opinion is necessary to confirm high grade dysplasia. Accurate staging of patients with oesophageal and gastric malignancy is critical to the development of an appropriate management plan. Oesophageal tumours are usually staged effectively with a combination of CT scanning of the chest and abdomen combined with endoscopic ultrasound scanning (in the absence of metastatic disease) and endoscopic ultrasound may be combined with fine needle aspiration cytology from the oesophageal tumour or adjacent lymph nodes. PET scanning may have a role in identifying patients with metastatic disease undetected by other imaging modalities and the results of further studies which will describe its precise role are awaited with much interest. MRI scanning, on the other hand, has established value in assessing the T and N stage of oesophagogastric cancers and may also be useful in the further characterisation of liver lesions. Endoscopic ultrasound scanning also has a role in the assessment of gastric cancers, particularly in patients with early gastric carcinoma and is useful in assessing the extent of carcinomatous infiltration while laparoscopy is particularly useful in patients with tumours below the diaphragm and may be combined with peritoneal cytology. The restaging of patients following initial treatment with chemotherapy or chemo-radiotherapy is less reliable, the distinction between tumour and fibrotic tissue being difficult on standard imaging techniques. PET scanning may have a role in assessing response. Much has been written, indeed very recently, on the initial staging of disease prior to direct therapeutic intervention and, recognising this, we refer the reader to the definitive texts and move, here, directly to a thorough consideration of the evidence base for direct clinical intervention in the investigation and management of gastro-oesophageal cancer.

In Chapter Four, the opening chapter of Part Two of the volume, Dickson, Rao, Chau and Cunningham review the place of peri-operative chemotherapy in oesophago-gastric cancer. As these authors discuss, oesophageal cancer is the sixth most common cause of cancer related mortality in the world and long-term survival remains poor, even for patients with localised disease. Surgery is considered the standard treatment, yet 5-year survival rates are below 20% for patients who undergo resection and this has led investigators to consider the value of peri-operative chemotherapy through several randomised studies. Interestingly, the two largest studies conducted to date have shown conflicting results. The UK Medical Research Council OE02 study demonstrated a survival benefit utilising preoperative 5FU and cisplatin compared with surgery alone whereas the US Intergroup study did not observe any survival difference. As a consequence of the results of these and other smaller studies, no international consensus yet exists for the use of preoperative chemotherapy in patients with localised carcinoma of the oesophagus and oesophagogastric junction, although it seems true to say that patients who achieve a clinical response and a pathological complete response have a better long-term outcome. The impact of perioperative chemotherapy in localised lower oesophageal and gastric cancer has recently been evaluated in a large randomised UK Medical Research Council study, the MAGIC trial. This compared, as Dickson and associates discuss, pre-operative and post-operative chemotherapy with 5-FU, epirubicin and cisplatin versus surgery alone, demonstrating that perioperative chemotherapy improves progression-free survival and increases resectability in operable lower oesophageal and gastric cancer with a trend towards improved overall survival that does not yet reach statistical significance. The use of biological markers in predicting patient response to therapy is currently generating much interest and functional imaging, molecular markers and gene expression profiling are all being evaluated to identify subgroups of patients who would benefit most from pre-operative treatment. Optimal integration of new cytotoxic drugs such as taxanes, irinotecan, oxaliplatin and oral fluoropyrimidines with molecularly targeted therapy may impact on the prognosis of gastro-oesophageal cancer in the future.

Oesophageal cancer is responsive to both chemotherapy and radiotherapy and multi-modality approaches strive to improve outcomes by addressing potential causes of treatment failure, although their impact is limited by the advanced stage of disease at presentation in most cases. Preoperative chemoradiation, as Crellin describes in Chapter Five, has shown variable results in trials. It does have the potential for increased toxicity and there may be a role for selected cases, particularly in squamous cancers, where disease is locally advanced and patients are otherwise fit, but the standard approach for resectable adenocarcinoma remains, overall, chemotherapy and surgery. The importance of a positive resection margin may also be addressed with post-operative radiotherapy, for which there is evidence of clinical significance in squamous carcinoma and a case may be made for a similar approach in patients with otherwise favourable prognosis adenocarcinoma. Increasingly, the focus for chemoradiation is in optimising definitive treatment as an alternative in patients who are unfit for, or choose not to undergo surgery. As Crellin makes clear, there is scope for improved activity with new drug combinations and radiotherapy techniques and the use of molecular predictors of response may allow patient selection for non-surgical approaches. In squamous cancers there are many questions which remain to be addressed in relation to the role of surgical resection, but controversy continues to surround the design of future trials. Nevertheless, there remains a role for radiotherapy alone, particularly in the elderly with very limited volume disease. New approaches to imaging, radiotherapy planning and treatment delivery should bring a better therapeutic ratio, but underline the need for rigorous quality assurance in future studies.

There is little doubt that the status of resection margins – including the circumferential margin – is an important part of the pathological assessment of many cancers and it is to an important consideration of the clinical significance of the circumferential margin that Mapstone turns in Chapter Six. Proximal and distal margins have traditionally been assessed in many tubular organs but the circumferential margin has frequently been ignored, despite increasing evidence that this parameter is important in the rectum for prognosis, correlation with radiology, assessing surgical technique and planning adjuvant treatment, although in the oesophagus the evidence is much less clear. Certainly, there is no evidence for margin involvement being important in planning treatment or any relationship with surgical technique and the evidence for its relevance to prognosis remains inconclusive. Mapstone nevertheless argues that this margin should still be assessed in all oesophageal, though not gastric, cancers. He points out that the international guidance for pathological staging of oesophageal cancers (along with all other cancers) has recently undergone major changes with some cancers to be upstaged, and some downstaged, by the new proposals – especially as they apply to assessing lymph node metastases, and Mapstone is clear in emphasising the need for standardisation and precision in pathological staging of these malignancies.

Resection remains the treatment of choice for patients with potentially curable gastric carcinoma and who are fit enough for surgery. Until recently there was no proven role for adjuvant chemotherapy, radiotherapy or synchronous chemo-radiotherapy in this context, but recently published meta-analyses now indicate that adjuvant chemotherapy of some sort provides a significant increase in overall survival and two recent post-operative adjuvant chemotherapy studies, based on fluorinated pyrimidines, have also shown a significant survival advantage when this therapy is given after a gastric cancer has been curatively resected. Adding to this evidence, as Hogg and co-authors discuss in Chapter Seven, there is now a large randomised study showing a significant survival benefit with post-operative adjuvant chemo-radiotherapy and while this study does perhaps have some defects in interpretation, mainly related to the completeness of the surgery, it was a well-constructed study with good radiotherapy quality control. The recently presented MAGIC study is also of no small significance, showing down-staging and increased resectability of gastric tumours, and while no overall survival benefit was found in this study, continued analysis of the data may yet reveal important effects. There is considerable debate as to the optimal surgical management for this group of patients and in particular, the extent of lymph node dissection. Two multi-centre trials from Europe have failed to demonstrate a survival benefit favouring D2 over D1 surgery for gastric carcinoma. In fact, the mortality following surgery was higher for the D2 resection groups in both trials. This may be partly due to the splenectomy and distal pancreatectomy, which was performed in addition to the D2 lymph node dissection in a number of patients. Despite these findings, the International Gastric Cancer Association Consensus (1997) favoured a D2 lymphadenectomy for patients with curable gastric cancer. There are therefore many questions that need to be answered. What is the best chemotherapy and when should it be given in relation to the surgery? Should chemoradiotherapy be advocated and what surgery should be adopted? Hogg et al believe that questions such as these could be answered by a national stomach trial enabling an adequate cohort of patients to undergo and complete all of the treatments, that is no too toxic to lead to treatment interruption and which is well supported by surgeons, radiotherapists and medical oncologists.

The improvements in survival that have accompanied the innovative approaches to therapy outlined thus far in the text are encouraging but they rarely result in cure. Our increased understanding of the biology of upper gastrointestinal malignancies in recent years has allowed the development of strategies targeting specific genetic changes in these tumours and it is to a stimulating review of this exciting area of research that Turner and Hochhauser turn in Chapter Eight. As the authors describe, the important but unsuccessful early trials targeted the processing (farnesylation) of the *ras* oncogene, which is mutated in virtually all pancreatic cancers, but subsequent studies have now identified a wide variety of other potential targets in tumours of the pancreas as well as, of course, oesophagogastric cancer. The ongoing research into such strategies will also need to take into account the stage of development of the cancer. For example, up-regulation of the cyclo-oxygenase 2 gene occurs early in progression to oesophageal cancer at the low grade dysplasia stage and COX-2 inhibitors would likely have benefit when used at that stage. Other therapies, such as inhibitors of the matrix metalloproteinases, would be used later in the disease pathway. Many candidate genes expressed in upper GI cancer have, as Turner and Hochhauser discuss, already been validated as therapeutic targets in other cancers, such as the epidermal growth factor receptor (EGFR), which is commonly upregulated in oesophageal cancer. The orally active quinazoline drug gefitinib has shown clinical benefit in non-small cell lung cancer and is now being tested in oesophago-gastric cancer. In addition, the antibody cetuximab, which blocks the EGFR ligand-receptor interaction, can sensitise irinotecan-resistant colonic tumours to irinotecan and will be of interest in therapy of upper gastrointestinal malignancies. The authors are clear that in future studies it will be critical to understand the basis for synergies between chemotherapy and strategies targeting the growth factor receptors given that this will then allow allow the design of appropriate combinations and schedules. Such combinations will allow inhibition of angiogenesis and metastasis which result in early dissemination of tumour cells.

We have dedicated Part Three of this volume to a detailed consideration of the evidence base for the management of pancreatic cancer. Key advances in the assessment and surgical treatment of pancreatic cancer have come from improvements in pre-operative assessment driven in the main by advances in imaging technology and postoperative care driven largely by a better understanding of the physiologic response to surgery and Mudan provides a thorough discussion of these developments in Chapter Nine. In most cases, as he describes, good quality CT will match good quality MR or EUS for diagnosis and the question of the small or indeterminate mass may be better clarified by EUS or PET scan. Staging of the primary tumour and of the nodal status is similarly matched with these imaging modalities but EUS opens the potential for pre-operative nodal sampling and of pre-operative locoregional or systemic therapy. Precise imaging of the regional vasculature is an important technical consideration in patient selection for operation. Indeed, most surgeons regard arterial involvement as an absolute contraindication for resection but venous involvement is a complicating factor rather than a contraindication. The precision of CT for vascular assessment is such that angiography is not required and modern CT-angiography software allows parity with MR angiography. Subtle cases, in particular of minor venous encasement, may benefit from linear Doppler-EUS to resolve. Small volume peritoneal disease remains impossible to detect by extracorporeal imaging. With the exception of the early pancreatic head primary or tumours of the ampulla evaluation of the peritoneal cavity by laparoscopy remains a helpful tool. As many as 20% of T3 tumours of the head and up to 50% of the pancreatic body harbour CT-occult intraperitoneal metastases. Moreover, laparoscopy for staging opens the potential for palliative bypass in selected inoperable cases.

The results from treating pancreatic ductal adenocarcinoma appear to be improving with increasing resection rates and reduced post-operative mortality reported by specialist pancreatic cancer teams. Developments with medical oncological treatments have been difficult, however, due to the fundamental aggressive biological nature of pancreatic cancer and the relative dearth of randomized controlled trials. Two recent trials of adjuvant therapy have changed our approach to treatment and have superseded the previous rather small studies. The GITSG trial was the first, smallest and only randomized trial from the USA. 43 patients all with clear resection margins (R0) were randomized to either surgery alone or surgery combined with 40Gy radiotherapy (with 5-FU radiosensitisation) and weekly 5-FU. The two-year survival rates were 42% and 15% respectively. The Norwegian trial randomized 47 patients to FAM chemotherapy or observation. No long-term survival benefit with chemotherapy was shown, but there was an improvement in median survival (23 months for chemotherapy *versus* 11 months for controls). The EORTC trial compared chemoradiotherapy with surgery alone in 218 patients with pancreatic or ampullary cancers. The survival improvement in the pancreas cancer group (median survival 17.1 months *versus* 12.6 months for observation) was not statistically significant.

There was no maintenance treatment with 5-FU. The ESPAC-1 trial with nearly 600 patients recruited overwhelms all other adjuvant trials in pancreatic cancer. 285 were entered into a 2x2 factorial design randomisation of chemotherapy *versus* no chemotherapy and radiotherapy *versus* no radiotherapy; the rest were randomised into a single option only. The median survival in patients receiving chemotherapy was significantly improved at 19.7 months compared with 14 months in the no chemotherapy group. The median survival of patients randomized to chemoradiotherapy was 15.5 months and is comparable to many other studies but was not different from those randomized to no chemoradiotherapy. The survival benefit of chemotherapy also applied to patients with R1 resection margins as well as those with R0 resection margins. Quality of life improved in all groups equally following surgery. Neither the type of resection nor the development of complications influenced the results of adjuvant treatment. For confirmation, the ESPAC-3 trial is randomizing patients to observation, 5-FU/FA as used in ESPAC-1 and gemcitabine. Exceptional progress has been made in the adjuvant treatment of pancreatic cancer in the last 10 years and the next decade is likely to witness even more remarkable developments. We have omitted a discreet chapter on adjuvant chemotherapy of pancreatic cancer in this volume, given the wealth of literature recently published elsewhere on this subject and we refer the reader to those sources for this information. Rather, we move now directly to a review of the current evidence base for the management of advanced disease.

Of the approximately 7000 people who are diagnosed in the UK annually with pancreatic cancer, approximately 5500 have advanced disease. The location of the tumour is likely to cause difficult symptoms, for example anorexia, abdominal pain, gastric outlet obstruction and weight loss and many patients require stenting for jaundice. Patients who receive no treatment have a median survival of around three months, but this can be improved with chemotherapy as evidenced by the results of trials where best supportive care was compared with drug therapy and also by the results of meta-analyses. However, even with modern therapy it is difficult to achieve a median survival beyond eight months. Gemcitabine, as Petty and Nicolson describe in Chapter Ten, was registered for use as a single agent as much for its palliating effect on symptoms (as measured by the composite scale of the Clinical Benefit Response) as for the survival benefit at 1 year (18% versus 2% for single agent bolus 5-fluorouracil). In the past few years, most clinical trials in advanced pancreatic cancer have compared gemcitabine alone with gemcitabine in combination with one or more drugs. There is to date no clear evidence of any benefit with combination therapy either using other chemotherapy drugs or 'biological' agents, but the national trial currently approved by the NCRN is a comparison of gemcitabine alone versus that plus capecitabine. Capecitabine is orally delivered and known to accumulate preferentially in the tumour as is seen in colorectal cancer. Data from one non-gemcitabine combination were published in 2003, and this Phase II study of 45 patients reported a median survival of 7 months with 29% 1-year survival using mitomycin-C, cisplatin and infusional 5-fluorouracil. The novel agent pemetrexed has a single agent activity of >20% in advanced pancreatic cancer and the phase III trial of gemcitabine with or without pemetrexed will report very shortly. It was estimated from one audit published in 2003 that only 7% of patients with advanced pancreatic cancer receive chemotherapy alone with 44% not receiving any treatment. This number needs to be increased if we are to offer the best therapy available for this difficult tumour. Although a rarer tumour, we have been concerned to include in this volume a discussion of the characteristics and management of biliary tract cancer and commend to colleagues Chapter Eleven by Armstrong and Valle which documents in no small detail our current knowledge and management of these particular tumours.

We have dedicated Part Four of the volume, the concluding Part, to a review of issues of importance to the clinical governance of upper gastrointestinal cancer services. A central 'plank' of the governance philosophy is the development and use of clinical guidelines which might guide local clinical practice. Upper GI cancer practice is, certainly, inundated with clinical guidelines. Indeed, worldwide there is huge variation in the quality of guidelines, which vary from statements of unsupported personal prejudice to well worked out documents based on systematic reviews of the literature. Within Europe an instrument has been developed (AGREE instrument) for the assessment of guidelines to determine whether they conform to an acceptable 'evidence-based' standard. In general, published UK guidelines are of a high standard and have a degree of acceptance internationally. They can be produced in the UK without general interference from interested groups, unlike the situation in the USA. Three principal groups of guidelines exist in upper GI cancer. Firstly, those from UK specialist societies (AUGIS, BSG, BASO), these include hepatocellular cancer (HCC), gastro-oesophageal cancer, cholangiocarcinoma, pancreatic cancer and colorectal liver metastases. Secondly, there are the Cochrane reviews, which include screening for HCC, lymphadenectomy and gastric cancer and pre-operative chemotherapy and chemo-radiotherapy in oesophageal cancer. Lastly, there is the DoH Upper GI cancer standards document. All have limitations in terms of application and utility. Firstly, guidelines must not be used as a gold standard for treatment but as a summary of evidence which may inform the treatment of an individual, that much is fundamental to notions of effective clinical practice. Also, the concept that a patient cannot be entered into a clinical trial which includes an arm not supported in a guidelines document should surely be resisted strongly. Secondly, guidelines are often incomplete because the evidence on which they are based cannot be derived from any clinical trial or, indeed, may be based on flawed trials – consider, in example, the UK D1/D2 gastrectomy trial. The need to continue to develop an evidence base for the effective management of upper gastrointestinal cancers therefore remains paramount.

Like much else in the modern NHS, changes in cancer service delivery have been at least in part driven by targets. While this has undeniably had some benefits for patients it has also exposed service deficiencies and underfunding. These deficiencies are currently being addressed in part by looking at processes such as the 'patient journey', with the aim of identifying so-called 'bottlenecks' and other inefficiencies in service delivery and additionally to highlight areas of good practice and innovation. The Cancer Collaborative, for example, has been instrumental in co-ordinating a mapping of the patient pathway and local cancer network meetings have proved in many cases effective in identifying and disseminating good practice. Examples include both shortened time between investigation/treatment and a better patient experience through upper GI cancer nurse specialists and better endoscopy waiting list management (list planning, backfilling of 'lost' lists, partial and full booking – to reduce DNA's –, common endoscopy waiting lists). Such initiatives are being rolled out across the country though the 'tool kit' piloted and promoted by the Endoscopy Modernisation project.

Initiatives such as dyspepsia clinics with urea breath testing or *H pylori* serology, based on recently revised BSG Dyspepsia guidelines (with NICE guidelines soon to follow) may free up endoscopy list space. The latter is critical, as while BSG surveys and presentations to the annual BSG meeting have shown that most units have been able to meet the 2 week wait targets for upper and lower GI cancer, this has been at the expense of 'routine' wait times for endoscopy and outpatients. 'Alarm' symptoms identify advanced cancers, but some patients do not present with alarm symptoms. Indeed, patients with 'early' and potentially curable cancers are more likely to present routinely because symptoms are not worrying. It is therefore crucial that routine wait times for endoscopy be kept short and it is of concern to those of us who believe that it is useful to identify and survey Barrett's oesophagus that fewer patients with uncomplicated reflux symptoms will be endoscoped if dyspepsia guidelines are widely followed.

The reconfiguration process for upper gastrointestinal malignancies is a challenge to the health economy managed by the Cancer Network. The Cancer Network's role in the reconfiguration process covers a number of distinct strands of work. The first is to co-ordinate the Peer Review process. Accredited and trained multi-disciplinary teams will visit each of the 34 English cancer networks. Their role is to test the preparedness of each of the NHS institutions in the network for the implementation of national guidance on commissioning. The second role of the network team is to ensure that the PCT commissioners are aware of their responsibility for prioritising the reconfiguration agenda against other cancer priorities for the financial year. The third role is to discuss with Chief Executives the need for patient and public involvement and possibly formal public consultation. Issues, which need to be tested, include the method by which a single centre is chosen to serve the needs of a population of 1.5 million for OG surgery and population of 3 million for pancreatic and biliary surgery. A fourth requirement is to understand the impact of cancer surgery for these tumours on non-cancer surgery. There is a 'knock-on' effect on the European Working Times Directive and postgraduate accreditation and training.

What other requirements for diagnostic and endoscopy work in those Trusts, which are no longer accredited for oesophagogastric surgery? To what extent will follow-up of patients take place in cancer units rather then the cancer centre? Approximately 90% of these patients will require either chemotherapy, radiotherapy or specialist palliative care. What are the workforce issues for the cancer centre and the cancer units respectively arising from an increase or a decrease in chemotherapy recommendations? A fifth requirement is to recognise that the majority of these patients will die of their disease and the majority are currently dying within acute sector beds. Is there any possibility of altering this policy through a more creative understanding of community, intermediate and Hospice care? All of these questions are to varying extents urgently in need of an answer and at the time of going to press of this volume, such questions have far from adequately been addressed or answered.

We conclude the book with two chapters which constitute Part Four, Chapter Twelve by Williams and Chapter Thirteen by Allum, the former describing the role of the Cochrane Collaboration in generating 'scientific' evidence for clinical decision making and the second reviewing the factors which have underpinned the re-organisation and re-provision of NHS services for the investigation and management of upper gastrointestinal cancers.

In the current age where doctors and health professionals are increasingly overwhelmed with clinical information, we have aimed to provide a fully current, fully referenced text which is as succinct as possible but as comprehensive as necessary. Consultants in Gastroenterology, Gastrointestinal Surgery and Medical and Clinical Oncology and their trainees are likely to find the volume of particular use as part of continuing professional development and specialist training respectively and we advance it specifically as an excellent tool for these purposes. We anticipate that the book will, in addition, prove invaluable to clinical nurse specialist and to oncology pharmacists and to the commissioners and planners of cancer services when in dialogue with their practising colleagues.

In conclusion we thank Lilly Oncology and Aventis Pharma for the grants of unrestricted educational sponsorship which helped organise a national symposium on the effective management of gastrointestinal cancer held with the British Society for Gastroenterology, The Royal College of Radiologists and the Association of Cancer Physicians at The Royal College of Physicians of London at which synopses of the constituent chapters of this volume were presented.

David Cunningham MD FRCP
Janusz Jankowski MD PhD FRCP
Andrew Miles MSc MPhil PhD

London, April 2005

Acknowledgements

The following colleagues contributed as members of the expert planning committee for the upper GI cancer project: Mr. William Allum, Professor David Cunningham, Professor Roger James, Dr. Robert Glynne-Jones, Dr. Daniel Hochhauser, Professor Jan Jankowski, Professor Andrew Miles, Dr. Marianne Nicolson, Dr. Mark Saunders, Mr. Jeremy Thompson. The contribution of Dr. Andreas Polychronis, SpR in Medical Oncology/Clinical Research Fellow, Imperial College at the Hammersmith Hospital, in the preparation of the current volume for publication, is also acknowledged.

PART 1

Epidemiology and genetics of upper gastrointestinal cancers

Chapter 1

The epidemiology of upper gastrointestinal malignancies: current perspectives and projections of disease burden

Clare Donnellan, David Forman and Simon Everett

Introduction

Upper gastrointestinal (GI) cancers are common throughout the world and have poor survival rates. They may be broken down into four types: oesophageal squamous carcinoma, oesophageal adenocarcinoma, gastric cardia adenocarcinoma and non-cardia (distal) gastric adenocarcinoma. These types have distinct epidemiological patterns and, where data allow, should be considered separately.

The incidence and mortality of the different subtypes of upper GI cancer are changing rapidly in most parts of the world and it can be assumed that potent environmental factors are responsible for this. Environmental triggers implicated include infection with *Helicobacter pylori* (*H. pylori*), smoking, alcohol intake, obesity, social deprivation and presence of gastro-oesophageal reflux disease. Some of these have a clear association (such as *H. pylori* with distal gastric cancer) but others are more hotly debated (such as the proposed link between *H. pylori* infection and reduced risk of adenocarcinoma of the oesophagus). There are some difficulties in interpreting some of the data because of incomplete registration of cancers and their subtypes. Nonetheless, further clarification of these risk factors may provide opportunities for cancer prevention in the future.

In this chapter we briefly summarise the available epidemiological data for the incidence and mortality of oesophago-gastric cancer worldwide. Many of the global data relate simply to gastric and oesophageal cancer, though there is a growing body of literature relating to the time trends of the four subtypes of upper GI cancer, so this will be summarised. Next, we review the data for the risk factors implicated in these time trends; finally we comment on predictions for the future, based on existing trends.

Incidence and mortality of upper gastrointestinal cancer
Stomach cancer

The most recent and comprehensive estimates of worldwide incidence and mortality from upper GI cancers have been provided by Parkin *et al.* (2001). It should be appreciated that these are only estimates; in 1990 only 42% of the world population was covered by registration systems producing incidence statistics on cancer. Worldwide, gastric cancer is now the third commonest malignancy (974,000 new cases per year in 2000) and is the second most common cause of death from cancer (10.4% of cancer deaths, 734,000 deaths annually), caused in part by very poor survival rates from this disease. There is significant global variation in incidence, with approximately two-thirds of cases occurring in developing countries. The highest incidence rates are in Japan, Central and South America, and Eastern Asia, though rates differ even within these areas. Lower rates are generally found in Africa. Despite declining incidence, stomach cancer is a significant contributor to global mortality, being the fourteenth commonest cause of all deaths in the world in 1990 (Murray & Lopez 1997).

UK data are derived from the 10 cancer registries in England and Wales and are compiled by The Office for National Statistics (ONS) (available on www.statistics.gov.uk). At the time of writing, the most recent complete data are for 2000, in which there were 7,865 new cases of stomach cancer in England (Cancer Statistics Registrations 2003). In 1997, gastric cancer in England and Wales ranked fifth in incidence in men and tenth in women (Quinn *et al.* 2002).

In all populations the incidence in males is approximately double that of females (Figure 1.1). The incidence of stomach cancer is higher in areas of social deprivation and there are significant ethnic variations, with rates in white people in the USA about half those in black people (Devesa *et al.* 1998). There is clearly a strong environmental component to the varying risk differences around the world: migrant populations from high-risk areas show a reduction of risk when they move to lower-risk areas (Kolonel *et al.* 1981), though the childhood environment appears to be particularly significant in determining risk (Coggon *et al.* 1990).

In the UK and worldwide, the incidence of stomach cancer has declined continuously in most countries over the past 50 years or more by approximately 1–4% per annum. In England and Wales, the age-standardised incidence of gastric cancer in men has decreased by 41% (from 31.8 to 18.9 per 100,000) and in women by 51% (from 15.1 to 7.3 per 100,000) between 1971 and 1998 (Newnham *et al.* 2003a) (Figure 1.2).

Survival from stomach cancer in England remains poor: based on patients diagnosed between 1990 and 1994, 1- and 5-year relative survivals were 30% and 14% for both sexes combined. Improvements in 5-year survival have been small, approximately 2% increase every 5 years, and UK survival lags significantly behind the European average (42% and 24%, 1- and 5 year survival, respectively) (Eurocare III study, unpublished data). One and 5-year survival rates are higher in women than men in all age groups (Newnham *et al.* 2003a).

Oesophageal cancer

Oesophageal cancer is the seventh most common malignancy worldwide and has the sixth highest cancer mortality rate, owing to poor survival rates. It accounts for

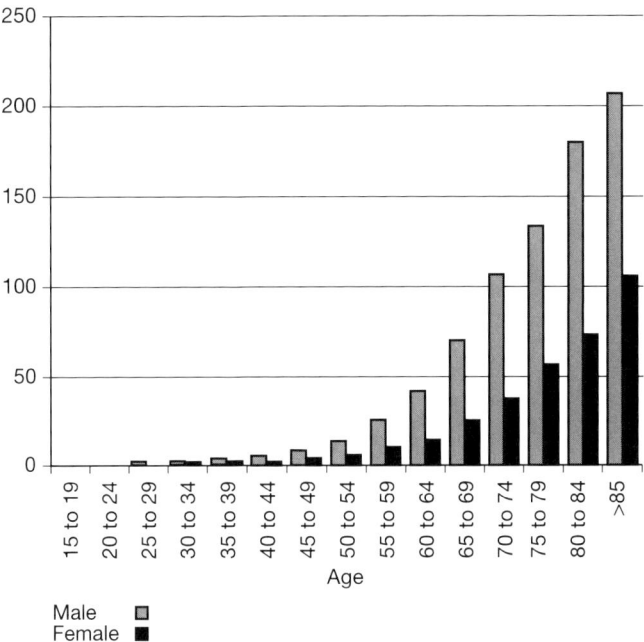

Figure 1.1 Gastric cancer incidence in England, 1999. Rates per 100,000 population of newly diagnosed gastric cancer in males and females according to 5-year age group. The overall age-standardised incidence rate per 100,000 population was 17.6 for males and 6.9 for females in England in 2000 (Cancer Statistics Registrations 2003).

355,000 deaths annually (5.4% of cancer deaths) (Parkin *et al.* 2001). Over 80% of cases occur in developing countries, but it has the greatest geographical variability of any cancer. Even within high risk areas, there are major variations in incidence, an effect seen most clearly in provinces of China. The countries with the highest incidence are in the Asian 'oesophageal cancer belt' (from northern Iran through the Central Asian republics to north–central China) plus East and Southeast Africa, eastern South America and parts of Western Europe (especially France and Switzerland). Again the incidence is generally higher in males (up to 6.5:1 male:female ratio in France) though there is variation in this ratio between geographical areas.

In England there were 6,033 new cases of oesophageal cancer diagnosed in 2000 (Cancer Statistics Registrations 2003). In 1997 the incidence of oesophageal cancer ranked seventh in men and thirteenth in women (Quinn *et al.* 2002). As with stomach cancer the incidence of oesophageal cancer at any one age is almost double for males than for females (Figure 1.3) and is commoner in areas of social deprivation. The age-standardised incidence increased in men by 67% (from 7.6 to 12.8 per 100,000) and

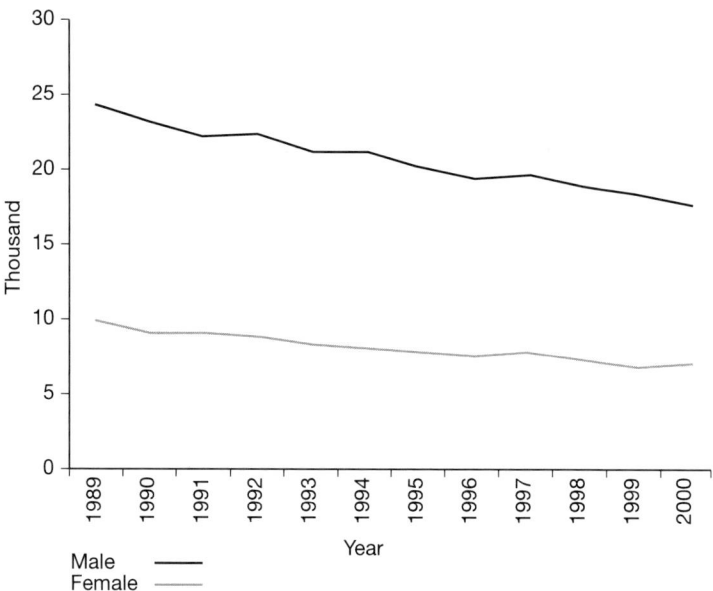

Figure 1.2 Gastric cancer incidence in England, 1989–1999. Data are directly age-standardised registration rates of gastric cancer per 100,000 population for males and females from 1989–2000 (Cancer Statistics Registrations 2002, 2003).

in women by 34% (from 4.2 to 5.7 per 100,000) between 1971 and 1998 (Newnham *et al.* 2003a) predominantly because of an increase in distal oesophageal adenocarcinoma (Figure 1.4). Nonetheless, gastric cancer was still commoner than oesophageal cancer in both men and women in 2000.

Survival from oesophageal cancer is also poor: for patients diagnosed between 1990 and 1994 in England, 1- and 5-year relative survival was 28% and 10% respectively for both sexes combined. For reasons that remain unclear, survival is consistently better in women than men, especially in younger age groups. Survival rates are lower than the average in Europe (33% and 10%, 1- and 5-year survival respectively), though the difference is less marked than for stomach cancer (Eurocare III study, unpublished data).

Time trends by morphological subtype

The pattern of upper GI cancer is changing rapidly around the world. In numerous case series and population based studies from America (Devesa *et al.* 1998), Canada Australia, New Zealand (Armstrong & Borman 1996) and several countries in Europe (Botterweck *et al.* 2000; Powell & McConkey 1990), there has been an increase in the incidence of adenocarcinoma of the distal oesophagus and/or gastric cardia (Figure 1.5). This increase began around the 1970s in both men and women, spanning all age

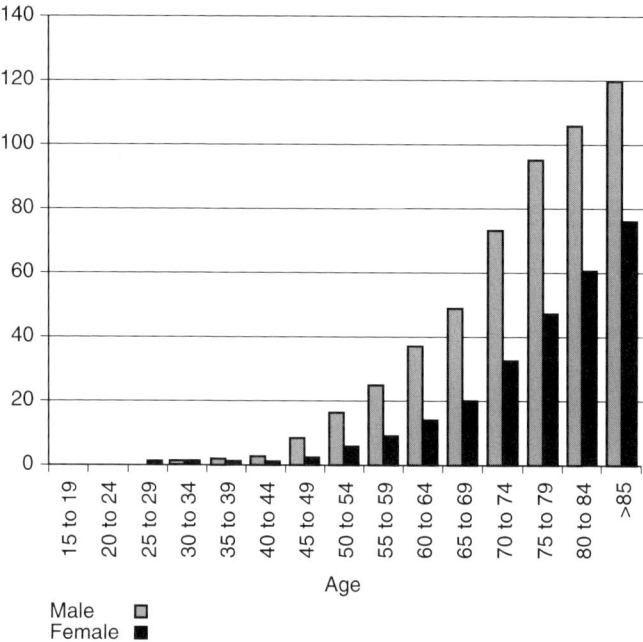

Figure 1.3 Oesophageal cancer incidence in England, 1999. Rates per 100,000 population of newly diagnosed oesophageal cancer in males and females according to 5-year age group. The overall age-standardised incidence rate per 100,000 population was 13.4 for males and 5.7 for females in England in 2000 (Cancer Statistics Registrations 2003).

groups, but is most pronounced in Caucasian men. The trend seems to be more marked in distal oesophageal adenocarcinoma than gastric cardia cancer, though it is possible that this is due to difficulties in classification and registration. There has probably been a similar rise in Barrett's oesophagus, generally considered the precursor to oesophageal adenocarcinoma, though the data are much more sparse (Conio *et al.* 2001).

In an important study using data available from the American National Cancer Institute's Surveillance, Epidemiology and End Results (SEER) program, Devesa *et al.* (1998) demonstrated a rise in the incidence of adenocarcinoma of the distal oesophagus by more than 350% between 1975 and 1995 in white American males, and the incidence surpassed that of squamous cell carcinoma in 1990. Parallel changes were seen in black males though oesophageal adenocarcinoma had much lower incidence than in white males and squamous cell carcinoma much higher. This meant squamous cell carcinoma remained much more common than oesophageal adenocarcinoma in black males in the 1990s. Similar, though less dramatic, increases were seen in gastric cardia cancer, which again was commoner in white males than

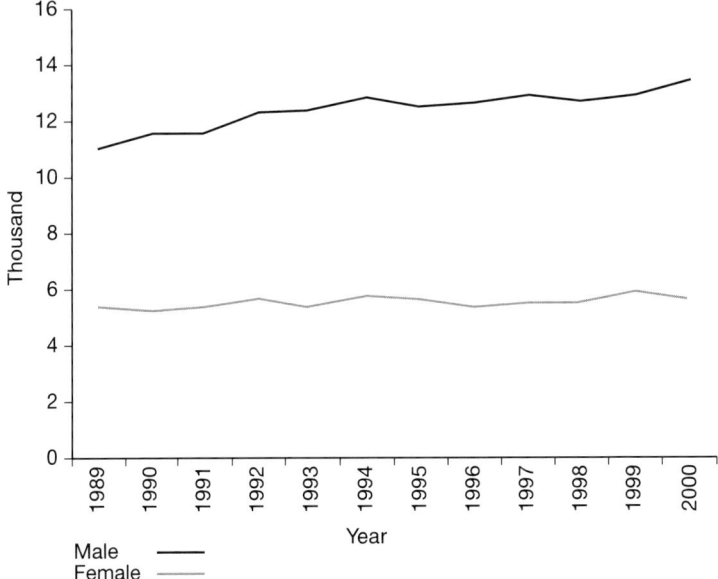

Figure 1.4 Oesophageal cancer incidence in England, 1989 to 1999. Data are directly age-standardised registration rates of oesophageal cancer per 100,000 population for males and females from 1989-2000 (Cancer Statistics Registrations 2002, 2003).

black males, whereas cancer of the distal stomach was commoner in black compared with white males, with a small decrease seen in white males only. By 1995 gastric cardia cancer was nearly as common as distal gastric cancer in white males but was much less common than distal cancer in black males. Thus, for black males the predominant disease remained distal gastric cancer and oesophageal squamous cell carcinoma, whereas for white males the upper GI cancer burden has changed from distal gastric adenocarcinoma and oesophageal squamous cancer to adenocarcinoma predominantly in the junctional region.

Similarly, in England and Wales, the age-standardised incidence of oesophageal squamous carcinoma in men has increased from 2.4 to 3.0 per 100,000 between 1971 and 1998. This is much less than the increase in the incidence of oesophageal adenocarcinoma over the same period (from 1.5 to 7.0 per 100,000), and this has now become the most common morphology in men. In women, however, the age-standardised incidence of oesophageal adenocarcinoma and squamous cell carcinoma have increased by similar amounts, from 0.4 to 1.5 per 100,000 and from 1.9 to 2.7 per 100,000 respectively, with squamous cell cancer remaining the more common morphology. Cardiac cancer has also shown similar, though less significant, changes in men and women (Newnham *et al.* 2003b; Solaymani Dodaran *et al.* 2001). Interestingly, the male:female ratio for oesophageal adenocarcinoma was 3.7:1 in

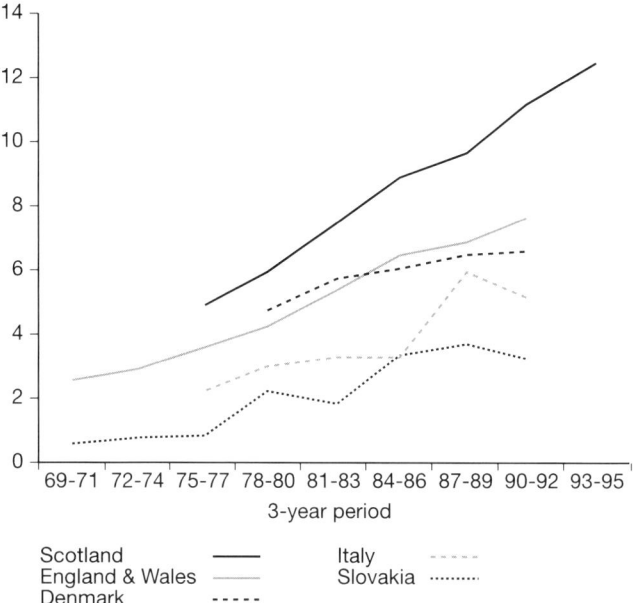

Figure 1.5 Incidence of adenocarcinoma of oesophagus and cardia in selected European countries (men). Age-standardised incidence rates per 100,000 population. Data are from selected countries in Europe: incidence did not increase significantly in France, Iceland, Switzerland and southern Ireland over a similar period (adapted from Botterweck *et al*. 2000).

1971 and has increased to 4.8:1 in 1998, whereas the sex ratio for squamous cell carcinoma has remained near unity (1.1:1). These striking observations and time trends in upper GI cancer subtype, particularly for gender and ethnic origin, remain inadequately explained.

These trends have been shown across several populations, but it is necessary to question the validity of some of these results. Between 1984 and 1993 more than 70% of upper GI cancers were recorded without subtype details in the Northern and Yorkshire cancer registry (Wayman *et al*. 2001). It is entirely possible, therefore, that the changes in the proportion of disease subtype can be explained by an over-registration of junctional type cancers as interest in this disease increases. Ekstrom *et al*. (1999) carefully classified all cases of gastric adenocarcinoma, according to subtype, between 1989 and 1994 and compared their results with the Swedish Cancer Registry. They found 98% of gastric cancers were included in the registry but that only 69% of cardia cancers were correctly classified and concluded that the true incidence of cardia cancer could be up to 45% higher or 15% lower than that reported in the Cancer Registry (Figure 1.6). Although the consistency of the rise in junctional cancers implies that this is a genuine effect, these data suggest that the magnitude of the change should be interpreted with considerable caution (Forman 2002).

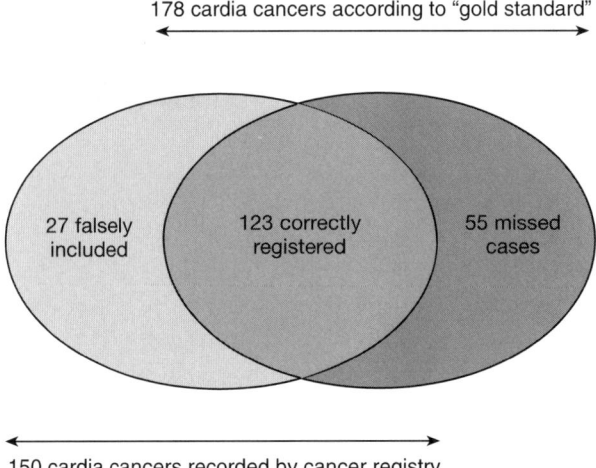

178 cardia cancers according to "gold standard"

| 27 falsely included | 123 correctly registered | 55 missed cases |

150 cardia cancers recorded by cancer registry

Figure 1.6 Gastric cardia cancer misclassification in Swedish cancer registry 1989–1994. A total of 178 cardia cancers were identified according to a 'gold standard' between 1989 and 1994 and compared with those registered with the Swedish cancer registry. Of 150 cancers recorded as cardia in the registry, only 123 were correctly registered (positive predictive value 123/150, 83%, completeness of registration 123/178, 69%) (Ekstrom *et al.* 1999).

Environmental agents

The rapid increases in gastric cardia cancer and oesophageal adenocarcinoma are dramatic and, with the above caveat, appear to be real. The explanation for these changes is unclear, though it seems highly probable that one or more environmental factors are responsible. Factors that have been implicated include dietary changes, reduction in *H. pylori* infection rates, improvements in social deprivation, changes in smoking and alcohol consumption and increasing incidence of obesity and gastro-oesophageal reflux disease. Clearly, some of these may be inter-related.

H. pylori infection

It is now well established that infection with *H. pylori* predisposes to distal gastric cancer (*Helicobacter* and Cancer Collaborative Group 2001) and the reduction in incidence of this disease may in part be explained by the reducing incidence of the infection (Banatvala *et al.* 1993; Roosendaal *et al.* 1997). Other significant factors include social and dietary changes, in particular the introduction of refrigeration with consequent reduction in salting and pickling of foods (Palli 1994).

Some authors have also suggested that the decline in *H. pylori* infection is responsible for an increase in gastro-oesophageal reflux disease, Barrett's oesophagus and distal oesophageal adenocarcinoma (Blaser 1999). The evidence for this has several different strands but remains circumstantial. Initially, it was observed in uncontrolled studies that eradication of *H. pylori* led to reflux symptoms in some patients (Labenz *et al.* 1997). Subsequently, case–control studies have reported a link between absence of *H. pylori* infection and presence of gastro-oesophageal reflux disease (Wu *et al.* 1999; Haruma *et al.* 2000; Raghunath *et al.* 2003). Further studies have suggested that *H. pylori* infection may protect by inducing corpus gastritis and reducing gastric acid output (Laheij *et al.* 2002). Two careful case–control studies have demonstrated that lower rates of infection with the more virulent strains of *H. pylori* (cagA positive) are related to increased rates of Barrett's oesophagus and oesophageal adenocarcinoma, though this effect was not evident if all *H.pylori* infections were included (Chow *et al.* 1998a; Vicari *et al.* 1998). Also, opposing time trends of distal gastric cancer and peptic ulcer disease (caused by *H. pylori*) on the one hand and reflux disease/Barrett's oesophagus/oesophageal adenocarcinoma on the other have led some to suggest that declining *H. pylori* infection rates may be a unifying factor responsible for all of these changes (El-Serag & Sonnenberg 1998).

However, these data do not prove causality and it is possible that an alternative explanation exists for this negative association. More recently, well-conducted randomised controlled trials have failed to demonstrate an increase in gastro-oesophageal reflux disease, either symptomatic or endoscopic, after eradication of *H. pylori*. This is true for patients with pre-existing gastro-oesophageal reflux disease (Moayyedi *et al.* 2001; Schwizer *et al.* 2001), non-ulcer dyspepsia (Moayyedi *et al.* 2000) and peptic ulcer disease (Malfertheiner *et al.* 2002). Finally, a meta-analysis of 12 nested case–control studies found no relation between *H. pylori* infection and gastric cardia cancer (*Helicobacter* and Cancer Collaborative Group 2001). It seems likely, therefore, that the negative association between *H. pylori* infection and oesophageal adenocarcinoma is not causal and alternative explanations must be sought for the rapid changes in incidence.

Deprivation

Numerous studies have shown that cancers of the stomach and oesophagus are more common in areas of greater deprivation, though deprivation in relation to subtype has been less well studied (Faggiano *et al.* 1997; Quinn *et al.* 2002). Furthermore, short-term survival from oesophageal and gastric cancer is marginally better in patients from less deprived areas, though this effect is not seen at 5 years and may, therefore, not relate to disease-specific factors (Newnham *et al.* 2003a). Results of studies examining the relation between incidence of cancers of the gastro-oesophageal junction and individual measures of deprivation have been inconsistent. However, Brewster *et al.* (2000) examined trends of upper GI cancer in Scotland in relation to deprivation using the Carstairs index, which is a composite determination of deprivation based on postcode area, between 1987 and 1996. Time trends in disease subtype were similar to those seen elsewhere in the UK. However, distal gastric cancer and oesophageal squamous cancer incidence were closely related to degree of deprivation, whereas incidence of oesophageal adenocarcinoma and gastric cardia cancer had no relation. These associations are difficult to understand: clearly deprivation has significant impact on other factors that are implicated in the aetiology of these tumours such as *H. pylori* infection rates, obesity and tobacco and alcohol use, and these relations will need to be teased out with further study.

Diet, smoking, alcohol, body mass index and gastro-oesophageal reflux disease

There have been numerous studies examining the relation between various risk factors and incidence of upper GI cancers. The studies in relation to cigarette smoking and alcohol use have been comprehensively reviewed by Wu *et al.* (2001). These studies vary considerably in terms of study size, design and population characteristics and frequently examine only single risk factors or single disease locations so can be difficult to interpret. However, three important population based case–control studies have recently been performed. These have been large, carefully conducted studies with clear definitions. Patients and their next of kin were interviewed for details of multiple factors that could impact on upper GI cancer incidence and statistical analyses controlled for confounding factors. Although they differ in some ways, together they provide a powerful insight into the aetiology of upper GI cancers in relation to these often inter-related risk factors.

The first study included 1143 subjects with all subtypes of upper GI cancer and 695 controls from three areas in the USA (Connecticut, New Jersey and Washington). They examined the effect of various factors on cancer incidence; namely smoking, alcohol, socio-economic status (Gammon *et al.* 1997), medication (Farrow *et al.* 1998), nutrient intake (Mayne *et al.* 2001), body mass index (Chow *et al.* 1998b) and gastroesophageal reflux disease (Farrow *et al.* 2000). The second study was a nationwide case–control study of the Swedish population, including 618 cases with oeosphageal adenocarcinoma, gastric cardia cancer or squamous cell carcinoma of the oesophagus (but not distal gastric cancer) and 820 controls. They studied smoking, alcohol use (Lagergren *et al.* 2000), body mass index (Lagergren *et al.* 1999a) and gastro-oesophageal reflux disease (Lagergren *et al.* 1999b) in relation to tumour location. The third study (Wu *et al.* 2001) was based on a multi-ethnic population in Los Angeles, USA. They compared smoking, alcohol intake and body size in 942 patients with adenocarcinoma of the oesophagus, gastric cardia and distal stomach to 1356 controls. They did not include patients with squamous cell carcinoma of the oeosophagus. The results of these three studies are summarised in Tables 1.1–1.4.

Smoking

Table 1.1 summarises the effect of smoking on cancer subtype. From these results it can be seen that smoking is probably a risk factor for all types of upper GI cancer.

Table 1.1 Risk of upper gastrointestinal cancer and cigarette smoking

Reference	Distal gastric cancer	Oesophageal adenocarcinoma	Gastric cardia cancer	Oesophageal squamous cell cancer
Gammon *et al*. (1997)	1.8 (1.2–2.7)	2.2 (1.4–3.3)	2.6 (1.7–4.0)	5.1 (2.8–9.2)
Lagergren *et al*. (2000)		1.6 (0.9–2.7)	4.5 (2.9–7.4)	9.3 (5.1–17.0)
Wu *et al*. (2001)	1.5 (1.1–2.2)	2.8 (1.8–4.3)	2.1 (1.5–3.1)	

Data are odds ratios (95% confidence intervals) for the risk of upper GI cancer in those who are current smokers versus those who have never smoked.

Table 1.2 Risk of upper gastrointestinal cancer and alcohol consumption

Reference	Distal gastric cancer	Oesophageal adenocarcinoma	Gastric cardia cancer	Oesophageal squamous cell cancer
Gammon *et al*. (1997)	0.8 (0.6–1.1)	0.7 (0.5–1.0)	0.7 (0.5–1.1)	3.5 (1.9–6.2)
Lagergren *et al*. (2000)		0.5 (0.3–0.9)	0.8 (0.5–1.2)	1.1 (0.6–2.1)
Wu *et al*. (2001)	1.0 (0.7–1.3)	0.7 (0.5–1.1)	1.0 (0.7–1.5)	

Data are odds ratios (95% confidence intervals) for the risk of upper GI cancer in those who drink alcohol versus those who have never drunk alcohol.

Table 1.3 Risk of upper gastrointestinal cancer and body mass index

Reference	Distal gastric cancer	Oesophageal adenocarcinoma	Gastric cardia cancer	Oesophageal squamous cell cancer
Chow *et al*. (1998)	1.2 (0.8–1.8)	2.9 (1.8–4.7)	1.6 (1.1–2.6)	0.6 (0.3–1.0)
Lagergren *et al*. (1999)		7.6 (3.8–15.2)	2.3 (1.5–3.6)	1.1 (0.7–1.9)
Wu *et al*. (2001)	1.0 (0.7–1.4)	1.9 (1.3–2.9)	1.6 (1.1–2.4)	

Data are odds ratios (95% confidence intervals) for the risk of upper GI cancer in those who have a BMI in the highest quartile versus those in the lowest.

Table 1.4 Risk of upper gastrointestinal cancer and gastro-oesophageal reflux symptoms

Reference	Distal gastric cancer	Oesophageal adenocarcinoma	Gastric cardia cancer	Oesophageal squamous cell cancer
Farrow *et al*. (2000)	1.4 (0.8–2.5)	5.5 (3.2–9.3)	1.2 (0.7–2.2)	0.5 (0.2–1.4)
Lagergren *et al*. (1999)		16.7(8.7–28.3)	2.3 (1.2–4.3)	1.4 (0.5–3.7)

Data are odds ratios (95% confidence intervals) for the risk of upper GI cancer in those who have daily reflux symptoms versus those who have none.

Generally, the effects of smoking were seen after controlling for potential confounders and were shown to be dose dependent in most cases. The effect of smoking is weakest for distal gastric cancer and the strongest relation is with squamous carcinoma, where Lagergren *et al.* (2000) reported a ninefold increased risk for current smokers compared with controls who had never smoked. The effect of smoking for junctional cancers is a little less consistent. The two American studies showed significant effects of smoking on gastric cardia and oesophageal adenocarcinoma with clear dose–responses. Lagergren *et al.* (2000) showed a significant effect of smoking on gastric cardia cancer but did not confirm the relation with oesophageal adenocarcinoma. Although the risk estimates were above unity, they were not statistically significant and showed no dose–response trends. The reason for this discrepancy is unclear but may relate to differences in case classification, population characteristics and study designs. Even so, a small effect of smoking is not ruled out by the Swedish study. It is notable that in the two American studies, the increased risk of smoking on junctional cancers was seen up to 20–30 years after cessation of smoking whereas the risk for squamous cell cancer dropped more rapidly, implying that, in these populations, smoking is an early event in the development of junctional cancers and recent changes in the incidence of smoking may not be reflected in current trends of cancer incidence.

Alcohol

The relation between cancer risk and alcohol consumption is more difficult to establish since different alcoholic beverages may confer different risks. However, it is apparent from Table 1.2 that alcohol has little impact on adenocarcinoma of the stomach or oesophagus. Although not clearly seen from the data in Table 1.2, which shows ever versus never consumption of any alcohol, there does appear to be an effect of alcohol on the development of squamous cell carcinoma of the oesophagus. The adjusted odds ratio (OR) for consuming any type of alcohol in the study by Gammon *et al.* (1997) was 3.5 (1.9–6.2) and this risk increased with rising levels of intake, reaching an OR of 7.4 (4.0–13.7) among those who consumed more than 30 alcoholic drinks per week. The risk of squamous oesophageal carcinoma was doubled in relation to use of beer and tripled in relation to use of liquor, whereas use of wine seemed to confer a small protection (OR 0.6, 0.4–0.9). In the Swedish study (Lagergren *et al.* 2000), alcohol did not confer a significant risk of squamous oesophageal carcinoma in users vs. non-users. However, significant risk was seen at the highest levels of alcohol consumption, especially for those who were both long-term smokers and heavy alcohol users (OR 23.1 (9.6–56.0) compared with never users).

Body mass index

Table 1.3 summarises the data relating to body mass index. All three studies reported similar findings: that increase in BMI does not affect risk of either distal gastric cancer or oesophageal squamous carcinoma, but that the risk of both gastric cardia adenocarcinoma and oesophageal adenocarcinoma were increased, the effect being greatest for oesophageal adenocarcinoma. The relation was dose-dependent in all three studies. Curiously, height was also inversely related to risk of oesophageal adenocarcinoma. The explanation for the increased risk of BMI on these cancers is unclear, though dietary factors may be relevant. Also, it is tempting to conclude that BMI acts as a surrogate marker for reflux disease; however, both Lagergren *et al.* (1999a) and Chow et *al.* (1998b) controlled for this and it is unlikely to be the major explanation. These important data imply that the rise in adult obesity in the Western world may in part explain the rapid increase in incidence of gastric cardia and oesophageal adenocarcinoma in the past 30 years.

Gastro-oesophageal reflux disease

The data in Table 1.4 demonstrate that gastro-oesophageal reflux disease is a potent risk factor for oesophageal and gastric cardia adenocarcinoma but does not play a role in distal gastric adenocarcinoma or oesophageal squamous cell carcinoma. Both Farrow *et al.* (2000) and Lagergren *et al.* (1999b) demonstrated significant dose-dependent relations between gastro-oesophageal reflux disease and oesophageal adenocarcinoma. This relation was independent of obesity, implying a likely causal relation. In both studies, the risk of oesophageal adenocarcinoma was greater for those with hiatal hernia, more frequent, more severe and longer-standing symptoms of reflux. For example, in the Swedish study the OR for oesophageal adenocarcinoma among persons with long-standing severe symptoms was 43.5 (95% confidence interval 18.3–103.5) and 4.4 (1.7–11.0) for gastric cardia adenocarcinoma. In both studies, the effect of reflux was larger for oesophageal adenocarcinoma than for gastric cardia cancer, and in the American study reflux was not seen to affect risk of cardia cancer at all. Nonetheless, these results suggest that, as with obesity, the dramatic rise in reflux disease in Western populations may account for a proportion of the rise in these cancers, though the explanation for the former remains unclear (El-Serag & Sonnenberg 1998).

Other factors

Use of acid-suppressive therapy has been associated with an increased risk of gastric cardia and oesophageal adenocarcinoma, though this may reflect their use for acid reflux disease (Farrow *et al.* 2000). There is good evidence that, as with colorectal cancer, regular intake of aspirin and other non steroidal anti-inflammatory drugs roughly halves the risk of all types of upper GI cancer, with the possible exception of gastric cardia cancer (Farrow *et al.* 1998). Dietary factors have been studied at length, especially for distal gastric cancer (Palli *et al.* 1994). In the three centre USA case–control study (Mayne *et al.* 2001), intake of fibre, beta-carotene, folate and vitamins C and B_6 were significantly and inversely associated with risk of all subtypes of upper GI cancer. In contrast, dietary cholesterol, animal protein and vitamin B_{12} were positively associated with all tumour types. The well-established link between dietary nitrite and distal gastric cancer was confirmed. Importantly, dietary fat was significantly associated with oesophageal adenocarcinoma even after controlling for body mass index and reflux symptoms.

Projections for the future

Projections of disease burden for the future have to take into account current trends of disease incidence and future changes in population demographics; they are therefore notoriously unreliable. The population of the world is increasing in size and age. Most of the population increase will be concentrated in the developing world in the next 50 years, whereas the proportion that are elderly in the developed world is predicted to increase from 14% to over 25% (Parkin *et al.* 2001). Urbanisation is likely to increase rapidly in the developing world, probably accompanied by urban poverty, whereas in the developed world rates of urbanisation are much less (Parkin *et al.* 2001). These factors are likely to have profound but rather unpredictable effects on cancer incidence around the world.

At current rates of population change the number of cases of gastric cancer worldwide will increase from 880,000 in 2000 to 2,440,000 in 2050 (Figure 1.7). For

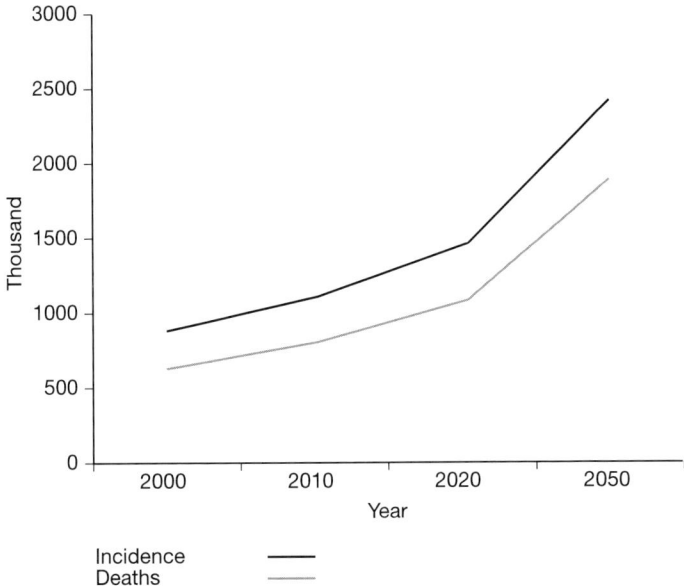

Figure 1.7 Gastric cancer: projected incidence and mortality (worldwide). Projected incidence and mortality of gastric cancer worldwide over the next 50 years. The most recent estimates of gastric cancer have been applied to the age- and sex-specific population projections for 2000, 2010, 2020 and 2050 but do not take into account underlying time trends. Adapted from Parkin *et al.* (2001).

Europe the predicted rise is more modest: from 190,000 to 300,000 new cases (Figure 1.8) (Parkin *et al.* 2001). However, these figures do not take into account the underlying downward trend for the incidence of gastric cancer. Should this continue at an annual decrease of 1% (as in the past decade), the projected number of new cases worldwide would be 900,000 in 2020 and 800,000 in 2050, i.e. similar to current numbers. Because survival has shown little sign of improvement, even in the developed world, then the number of deaths from gastric cancer is unlikely to be much less than the incidence and gastric cancer will remain a significant public health burden. Unfortunately, the assumption that current trends will continue unchanged for the next 50 years is likely to prove incorrect: as recent decades have shown, major changes in cancer incidence can occur abruptly and unpredictably. Indeed the above projection does not take into account the recent rise in oesophageal cancer, especially adenocarcinoma, which is likely to overtake gastric cancer as a cause of death in areas of the Western world in the near future (Newnham *et al.* 2003b).

Conclusions

Upper GI cancers are common diseases with high mortality both in the UK and worldwide. The most striking feature of these cancers is the rapid change in incidence

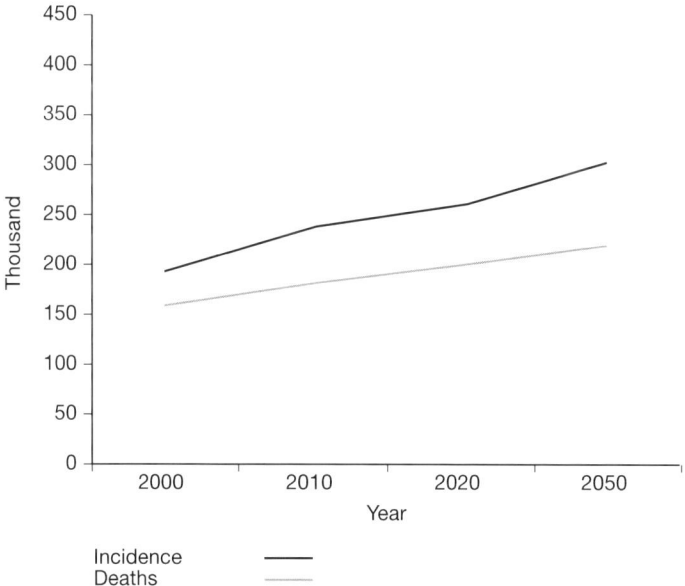

Figure 1.8 Gastric cancer: projected incidence and mortality (Europe). Projected incidence and mortality of gastric cancer in Europe over the next 50 years. The most recent estimates of gastric cancer have been applied to the age- and sex-specific population projections for 2000, 2010, 2020 and 2050 but do not take into account underlying time trends. Adapted from Parkin *et al.* (2001).

of disease subtypes, characterised by an increase in adenocarcinoma of the gastric cardia and distal oesophagus and a decrease in distal gastric cancer, especially in white caucasian males. Recent large epidemiological studies have suggested causes for these changes, most notably an increase in obesity and gastro-oesophageal reflux disease, though the underlying reason for the latter is more difficult to establish. Further research into preventative measures for these diseases is important as improvements in survival have been negligible and projections suggest that these diseases will remain important causes of death worldwide well into this century.

References

Armstrong, R. W. & Borman, B. (1996). Trends in incidence rates of adenocarcinoma of the oesophagus and gastric cardia in New Zealand, 1978–1992. *International Journal of Epidemiology* **25**, 941–947.

Banatvala, N., Mayo, K., Megraud, F., Jennings, R., Deeks, J. J. & Feldman, R. A. (1993). The cohort effect and *Helicobacter pylori*. *Journal of Infectious Diseases* **168**, 219–221.

Blaser, M. J. (1999). Hypothesis: the changing relationships of *Helicobacter pylori* and humans: implications for health and disease. *Journal of Infectious Diseases* **179**, 1523–1530.

Botterweck, A. A. M., Schouten, L. J., Volovics, A., Dorant, E. & van den Brandt, P. (2000). Trends in incidence of adenocarcinoma of the oesophagus and gastric cardia in ten European countries. *International Journal of Epidemiology* **29**, 645–654.

Brewster, D. H., Fraser, L. A., McKinney, P. A. & Black, R. J. (2000). Socioeconomic status and risk of adenocarcinoma of the oesophagus and cancer of the gastric cardia in Scotland. *British Journal of Cancer* **83**, 387–390.

Cancer Statistics Registrations (2002). Registrations of cancer diagnosed in 1998, England. Series MB1 No. 29. London: Office of National Statistics.

Cancer Statistics Registrations (2003). Registrations of cancer diagnosed in 2000, England. Series MB1 No. 31. London: Office of National Statistics.

Chow, W.-H., Blaser, M. J., Blot, W. J., Gammon, M. D., Vaughan, T. L., Risch, H. A., Perez-Perez, G. I., Schoenberg, J. B., Stanford, J. L., Rotterdam, H., West, A. B. & Fraumeni, J. F. Jr (1998a). An inverse relation between cagA+ strains of *Helicobacter pylori* infection and risk of esophageal and gastric cardia adenocarcinoma. *Cancer Research* **58**, 588–590.

Chow, W.-H., Blot, W. J., Vaughan, T. L., Risch, H. A., Gammon, M. D., Stanford, J. L., Dubrow, R., Schoenberg, J. B., Mayne, S. T., Farrow, H. A., West, A. B., Rotterdam, H., Niwa, S. & Fraumeni, J. F. Jr (1998b). Body mass index and risk of adenocarcinomas of the esophagus and gastric cardia. *Journal of the National Cancer Institute* **90**, 150–155.

Coggon, D., Osmond, C. & Barker, D. J. (1990). Stomach cancer and migration within England and Wales. *British Journal of Cancer* **61**, 573–574.

Conio, M., Cameron, A. J., Romero, Y., Branch, C. D., Schleck, C. D., Burgart, L. J., Zinsmeister, A. R., Melton, L. J. III & Locke, G. R. III (2001). Secular trends in the epidemiology and outcome of Barrett's oesophagus in Olmsted County, Minnesota. *Gut* **48**, 304–309.

Devesa, S. S., Blot, W. J. & Fraumeni, J. F. Jr (1998). Changing patterns in the incidence of esophageal and gastric carcinoma in the United States. *Cancer* **83**, 2049–2053.

Ekstrom, A. M., Signorello, L. B., Hansson, L.-E., Bergstrom, R., Lindgren, A. & Nyren, O. (1999). Evaluating gastric cancer misclassification: a potential explanation for the rise in cardia cancer incidence. *Journal of the National Cancer Institute* **91**, 786–90.

El-Serag, H.B. & Sonnenberg, A. (1998). Opposing time trends of peptic ulcer and reflux disease. *Gut* **43**, 327–333.

Faggiano, F., Partanen, T., Kogevinas, M. & Boffetta, P. (1997). Socioeconomic differences in cancer incidence and mortality. In *Social Inequalities and Cancer* (ed. M. Kogevinas, N. Pearce, M. Susser & P. Boffetta), pp. 65–176. IARC Scientific Publication No. 138. Lyon: International Agency for Research on Cancer.

Farrow, D. C., Vaughan, T. L., Hansten, P. D., Stanford, J. L., Risch, H. A., Gammon, M. D., Chow, W. H., Dubrow, R., Ahsan, H., Mayne, S. T., Schoenberg, J. B., West, A. B., Rotterdam, H., Fraumeni, J. F. Jr & Blot, W. J. (1998). Use of aspirin and other nonsteroidal anti-inflammatory drugs and risk of esophageal and gastric cancer. *Cancer Epidemiology, Biomarkers and Prevention* **7**, 97–102.

Farrow, D. C., Vaughan, T. L., Sweeney, C., Gammon, M. D., Chow, W. H., Risch, H. A., Stanford, J. L., Hansten, P. D., Mayne, S. T., Schoenberg, J. B., Rotterdam, H., Ahsan, H., West, A. B., Dubrow, R., Fraumeni, J. F. Jr & Blot, W. J. (2000). Gastroesophageal reflux disease, use of H_2 receptor antagonists, and risk of esophageal and gastric cancer. *Cancer Causes and Control* **11**, 231–238.

Forman, D. (2002). Counting cancers at the junction – a problem of routine statistics. *European Journal of Gastroenterology and Hepatology* **14**, 99–101.

Gammon, M. D., Schoenberg, J. B., Ahsan, H., Risch, H. A., Vaughan, T. L., Chow, W.-H., Rotterdam, H., West, A. B., Dubrow, R., Stanford, J. L., Mayne, S. T., Farrow, D. C., Niwa, S., Blot, W. J., Fraumeni, J. F. Jr (1997). Tobacco, alcohol, and socioeconomic status and adenocarcinomas of the esophagus and gastric cardia. *Journal of the National Cancer Institute* **89**, 1277–1284.

Haruma, K., Hamada, H., Mihara, M., Kamada, T., Yoshihara, M., Sumii, K., Kajiyama, G. & Kawanishi, M. (2000). Negative association between *Helicobacter pylori* infection and reflux esophagitis in older patients: case–control study in Japan. *Helicobacter* **5**, 24–29.

Helicobacter and Cancer Collaborative Group (2001). Gastric cancer and *Helicobacter pylori*: a combined analysis of 12 case control studies nested within prospective cohorts. *Gut* **49**, 347–353.

Kolonel, L. N., Nomura, A. M., Hirohata, T., Hankin, J. H. & Hinds, M. W. (1981). Association of diet and place of birth with stomach cancer incidence in Hawaii Japanese and Caucasians. *American Journal of Clinical Nutrition* **34**, 2478–2485.

Labenz, J., Blum, A. L., Bayerdorffer, E., Meining, A., Stolte, M. & Borsch, G. (1997). Curing *Helicobacter pylori* infection in patients with duodenal ulcer may provoke reflux oesophagitis. *Gastroenterology* **112**, 1442–1447.

Lagergren, J., Bergstrom, R. & Nyren, O. (1999a). Association between body mass and adenocarcinoma of the esophagus and gastric cardia. *Annals of Internal Medicine* **130**, 883–890.

Lagergren, J., Bergstrom, R., Lindgren, A. & Nyren, O. (1999b). Symptomatic gastroesophageal reflux as a risk factor for esophageal adenocarcinoma. *New England Journal of Medicine* **340**, 825–831.

Lagergren, J., Bergstrom, R., Lindgren, A. & Nyren, O. (2000). The role of tobacco, snuff and alcohol use in the aetiology of cancer of the oesophagus and gastric cardia. *International Journal of Cancer* **85**, 340–346.

Laheij, R. J. Van Rossum, L. G., De Boer, W. A. & Jansen, J. B. (2002). Corpus gastritis in patients with endoscopic diagnosis of reflux oesophagitis and Barrett's oesophagus. *Alimentary Pharmacology and Therapeutics* **16**, 887 891.

Malfertheiner, P., Dent, J., Zeijlon, L., Sipponen, P., Veldhuyzen Van Zanten, S. J. O., Burman, C.-F., Lind, T., Wrangstadh, M., Bayerdorffer, E. & Lonovics, J. (2002). Impact of

Helicobacter pylori eradication on heartburn in patients with gastric or duodenal ulcer disease – results from a randomized trial programme. *Alimentary Pharmacology and Therapeutics* **16**, 1431–1442.

Mayne, S. T., Risch, H. A., Dubrow, R., Chow, W.-H., Gammon, M. D., Vaughan, T. L., Farrow, D. C., Schoenberg, J. B., Stanford, J. L., Ahsan, H., West, A. B., Rotterdam, H., Blot, W. J. & Fraumeni, J. F. Jr (2001). Nutrient intake and risk of subtypes of esophageal and gastric cancer. *Cancer Epidemiology, Biomarkers and Prevention* **10**, 1055–1062.

Moayyedi, P., Feltbower, R., Brown, J., Mason, S., Mason, J., Nathan, J., Richards, I. D. G., Dowell, A. C. & Axon, A. T. R. (2000). Effect of population screening and treatment for *Helicobacter pylori* on dyspepsia and quality of life in the community: a randomised controlled trial. *The Lancet* **355**, 1665–1669.

Moayyedi, P., Bardhan, C., Young, L., Dixon, M. F., Brown, L. & Axon, A. T. R. (2001). *Helicobacter pylori* eradication does not exacerbate reflux symptoms in gastroesophageal reflux disease. *Gastroenterology* **121**, 1120–1126.

Murray, C. J. L. & Lopez, A. D. (1997). Mortality by cause for eight regions of the world: Global Burden of Disease Study. *The Lancet* **349**, 1269–1276.

Newnham, A., Quinn, M. J., Babb, P., Kang, J. Y. & Majeed, A. (2003a). Trends in oesophageal and gastric cancer incidence, mortality and survival in England and Wales 1971–1998/1999. *Alimentary Pharmacology and Therapeutics* **17**, 655–664.

Newnham, A., Quinn, M. J., Babb, P., Kang, J. Y. & Majeed, A (2003b). Trends in the subsite and morphology of oesophageal and gastric cancer in England and Wales 1971–1998. *Alimentary Pharmacology and Therapeutics* **17**, 665–676.

Palli, D. (1994). Dietary factors. *European Journal of Gastroenterology and Hepatology* **6**, 1076–1082.

Parkin, D. M., Bray, F. I. & Devesa, S. S. (2001). Cancer burden in the year 2000. The global picture. *European Journal of Cancer* **37**, S4–S66.

Powell, J. & McConkey, C. C. (1990). Increasing incidence of adenocarcinoma of the gastric cardia and adjacent sites. *British Journal of Cancer* **62**, 440–443.

Quinn , M., Babb, P., Brock, A., Kirby, L. & Jones, J. (2002). Office for National Statistics. Cancer Trends in England and Wales 1950–1999. London: The Stationery Office.

Raghunath, A., Hungin, A. P. S., Wooff, D. & Childs, S. (2003). Prevalence of *Helicobacter pylori* in patients with gastro-oesophageal reflux disease: systematic review. *British Medical Journal* **326**, 737–739.

Roosendaal, R., Kuipers, E. J., Buitenwerf, J., van Uffelen, C., Meuwissen, S. G., van Kamp, G. J., Vandenbroucke-Grauls, C. M. (1997). *Helicobacter pylori* and the birth cohort effect: evidence of a continuous decrease of infection rates in childhood. *American Journal of Gastroenterology* **92**, 1480–1482.

Schwizer, W., Thumshim, M., Dent, J., Guldenschuh, I., Menne, D., Cathomas, G. & Fried, M. (2001). *Helicobacter pylori* and symptomatic relapse of gastro-oesophageal reflux disease: a randomised controlled trial. *The Lancet* **357**, 1738–1742.

Solaymani Dodaran, M., Silcocks, P. B. & Logan, R. F. A. (2001). Continuing rise in incidence of oesophageal adenocarcinoma in England and Wales. *Gut* **48** (Suppl. 1), 30A (abstract).

Vicari, J. J., Peek, R. M., Falk, G. W., Goldblum, J. R., Easley, K. A., Schnell, J., Perez-Perez, G. I., Halter, S. A., Rice, T. W., Blaser, M. J. & Richter, J. E. (1998). The seroprevalence of cagA-positive *Helicobacter pylori* strains in the spectrum of gastroesophageal reflux disease. *Gastroenterology* **115**, 50–57.

Wayman, J., Forman, D. & Griffin, S. M. (2001). Monitoring the changing pattern of esophago-gastric cancer: data from a UK cancer registry. *Cancer Causes and Control* **12**, 943–949.

Wu, A.H., Wan, P. & Bernstein, L. (2001). A multiethnic population-based study of smoking, alcohol and body size and risk of adenocarcinomas of the stomach and esophagus (United States). *Cancer Causes and Control* **12**, 721–732.

Wu, J. C., Sung, J. J., Ng, E. K., Go, M. Y., Chan, W. B., Chan, F. K., Leung, W. K. & Choi, C. L. (1999). Chung SC. Prevalence and distribution of *Helicobacter pylori* in gastroesophageal reflux disease: a study from the East. *American Journal of Gastroenterology* **94**, 1790–1794.

Chapter 2

The genetics of upper gastrointestinal malignancy

Rebecca C. Fitzgerald and Carlos Caldas

Introduction

The new high-throughput technologies available to us mean that rapid advances are being made in genetics. Furthermore, these advances are beginning to have an impact on our management of those upper gastrointestinal (GI) cancers with a clearly defined inherited genetic basis. It will be some time before we understand the role of inherited susceptibility to the more common, sporadic cancers. In addition, although we have a reasonable understanding of the accumulation of somatic genetic mutations in the GI tissue itself during carcinogenesis, this has not yet altered clinical management. In the future, genetics has the potential to revolutionise our ability to detect patients at risk for cancer development and to classify tumours more accurately.

In this chapter the advances in our understanding of (1) the role of inherited susceptibility, and (2) the accumulation of somatic genetic mutations in the target tissues during carcinogenesis, will be illustrated by reference to oesophago-gastric tumours.

Cancer-related germline mutations: high- and low-penetrance genes

There is increasing evidence that there is an inherited component to many of the common cancers (Easton & Peto 1990), and upper GI cancers are no exception. One of the greatest contemporary advances in biomedical research is the identification of germline (heritable) gene mutations associated with cancer. Testing for cancer-related gene mutations can identify individuals at high risk of disease. The aim of this exercise is to help the affected individuals to reduce their own cancer risk (if preventive measures are available) and hence to reduce the burden of cancer. However, it should be remembered that the contribution of inherited susceptibility genes to cancer outcomes for a given population will be very variable. The outcomes will be determined by the degree of penetrance of that gene (i.e. the proportion of carriers of a mutant allele who express the disease associated with that mutation, which will vary from high to low), the effect of other modifying genes and the contribution of environmental influences. From a practical point of view, high-penetrance genes that cause family cancer syndromes can have a substantial impact in affected families, but they only affect a small proportion of the population.

In contrast, cancer susceptibility genes with lower penetrance contribute to common sporadic cancers and thus affect a larger segment of the population. In the case of low-penetrance genes, multiple genes tend to interact with each other to increase the risk and environmental effects contribute significantly to the disease manifestation.

High-penetrance genes and upper gastrointestinal cancers

A small percentage of oesophago-gastric cancers occur as a result of clearly identified cancer predisposition syndromes (summarised in Table 2.1). The two-hit theory of Knudson (Knudson 1985) predicts that in familial cancer syndromes the genotype of each neoplasm is determined by the presence of the inherited allele with a germline mutation and by the loss of the corresponding wild-type allele through allelic deletion. In some cases, such as hereditary diffuse gastric cancer, the specific gene responsible has been identified. It is also likely that high-penetrance susceptibility genes account for some of the observed familial clustering for which a single genetic locus has not yet been identified. In such cases, the relative risk increases markedly when the age of the index case decreases or the number of affected individuals in a cluster increases.

Hereditary cancer syndromes

Squamous oesophageal cancer and tylosis

The association between the skin disorder tylosis (focal non-epidermolytic palmoplantar keratoderma; NEPPK) and squamous oesophageal carcinoma is well documented. Tylosis is an autosomal dominant disorder of the skin that manifests as focal thickening of the palmar and plantar surfaces together with oral lesions and shows complete penetrance by the age of twenty. The risk of a UK family member with tylosis developing an oesophageal cancer is 90% by the age of 70 (Ellis *et al.* 1993), whereas the relative risk for US family members is 37 ($p < 0.00001$). The incidence of other common cancers in these families is not altered compared with the normal Caucasian population. The causative locus has been designated the tylosis oesophageal cancer (TOC) gene and has been localised to a small region (0.5 Mb) on chromosome 17q25, proximal to the type 1 keratin gene cluster. However, this region of chromosome 17q25 is relatively gene rich and is predicted to encode for between 13 and 50 genes and the TOC locus remains elusive (Risk *et al.* 2002). In addition to its role in autosomal dominantly inherited squamous oesophageal cancer, recent studies on the loss of heterozygosity have implicated the TOC gene in sporadic squamous cell carcinoma and Barrett's adenocarcinoma (Risk *et al.* 1999).

Multiple leiomyomas of the upper gastrointestinal tract

Multiple leiomyomas of the upper GI tract (oesophagus, stomach and duodenum) occur in multiple endocrine neoplasia type 1 (MEN-1) is an autosomal dominant hereditary disorder characterised by multiple parathyroid, pancreatic, duodenal and pituitary neuroendocrine tumours. The duodenal tumours are usually gastrinomas, which may be small and multiple. These gastrinomas are not associated with high gastrin levels until the tumour burden is advanced and they do have a high tendency to metastasise to the regional lymph nodes. Whereas symptoms due to acid hypersecretion can be effectively treated with proton pump inhibitors, surgery will rarely cure gastrinoma patients with MEN-1 syndrome. However, early surgical intervention with distal pancreatectomy and duodenotomy may significantly reduce the tumour burden and prolong survival (Thompson 1998). It has recently been demonstrated that leiomyomata of the oesophagus arise as independent clones as a result of MEN1 gene alterations and hence they should be considered as an integral part of the MEN1 sydrome (McKeeby *et al.* 2001).

Neuroendocrine and some mesenchymal tumours associated with MEN-1 have documented gene alterations on chromosome 11q13 (Larsson *et al.* 1988; Chandrasekharappa *et al.* 1997). It is currently recommended that genetic screening of relatives should be performed and those with positive genetic test results are then offered annual screening with tumour markers (e.g. chromogranin A or pancreatic polypeptide). Malignancy can generally be expected to occur between 10 and 30 years after the onset of biochemically detectable pancreatic disease. Thus, pancreatic surgery may help to gain substantial periods without malignant development (Skogseid *et al.* 1996; Dean *et al.* 2000).

Barrett's adenocarcinoma

There are several case reports of families with multiple affected persons with heartburn, Barrett's oesophagus and sometimes adenocarcinoma in up to four generations (Romero & Locke 1999). Analysis of the pedigrees in these studies suggests an autosomal dominant pattern of inheritance with incomplete penetrance. However, so far, candidate gene(s) have not been identified; part of the difficulty lies in the ascertainment of large pedigrees.

Hereditary diffuse gastric cancer

Hereditary diffuse gastric cancers (HDGCs) are the histopathological subtype sometimes referred to as linitis plastica. A subset of these diffuse type cancers (1–2% per cent of all gastric cancers) are hereditary, and recently linkage analysis has implicated E-cadherin (CDH1) mutations in an estimated 25% of them (Guilford *et al.* 1998). Because E-cadherin is a cell-adhesion molecule, it is thought that mutations in CDH1 may lead to the diffuse phenotype as a result of aberrant cell–cell adhesion. Most of the genetic abnormalities reported in CDH1 are inactivating mutations (splice-site, frameshift and non-sense) rather than missense and they are evenly distributed along the E-cadherin gene. *CDH-1* is a tumour suppressor gene and hence loss or inactivation of the remaining normal allele would be expected to be a required event in susceptible individuals with a germline mutation. The 'second hit' is normally deletion of the whole gene or else silencing of the promoter region of the gene by methylation (Berx *et al.* 1998; Grady *et al.* 2000).

Research on these families has also shown that penetrance of the *CDH1* gene is high, with an estimated range of 70–80%. In other words, if you carry the abnormal E-cadherin gene you have a 70–80% lifetime risk of developing gastric cancer (Pharoah *et al.* 2001). This high penetrance is similar to the risk for breast cancer in *BRCA1* carriers.

The clinical consequences of this work are far-reaching (Fitzgerald & Caldas 2002). The identification of the gene has resulted in the uptake of genetic screening by asymptomatic individuals in affected families. Families are keen to have the genetic testing performed because of the highly lethal nature of HDGC. However, the optimal clinical management strategy is not clear. The therapeutic options currently available are either endoscopic surveillance for detecting early, curable gastric cancers or else a prophylactic gastrectomy. So far, two groups (Chun *et al.* 2001; Huntsman *et al.* 2001) have shown that prophylactic resected stomachs from different families all carried a multifocal signet ring cancer. Importantly, surveillance using endoscopy and multiple biopsies had failed to identify intramucosal carcinoma in all of the surveilled cases. Further studies and longer-term follow-up are needed to determine whether prophylactic gastrectomy extends life expectancy and whether there is an increased incidence of cancers at other sites (e.g. breast (Berx *et al.* 1995; Keller *et al.* 1999) and colonic (Richards *et al.* 1999)). Another important research question is whether surveillance can be improved so that prophylactic surgery can be obviated.

The gene(s) responsible for the remaining 40–75% of hereditary diffuse gastric cancers which are not accounted for by mutations in CDH1 still remain to be identified.

Familial syndromes associated with small intestinal neoplasms

There are several familial syndromes associated with small intestinal tumours which may be benign or malignant (summarised in Table 2.1). The commonest of these are familial adenomatous polyposis (FAP), Peutz–Jeghers syndrome and neuro-fibromatosis Type 1. All of these syndromes raise questions about genetic testing for asymptomatic individuals and the optimal management strategy.

The colon is generally at greatest risk for malignancy in these syndromes, and prophylactic colectomy is recommended depending upon the lifetime risk for colorectal cancer in that syndrome and in that specific family. A major problem in these syndromes such as FAP and Gardner's syndrome is the management of the risk for duodenal cancers. This is complicated by the fact that although over 95% of patients have identifiable polyps only 5% go on to develop cancer (Nugent *et al.* 1993). Therefore, clinical surveillance is generally recommended. A grading system (Spigelman system) has been developed to stratify the risk for cancer development

Table 2.1 Familial syndromes associated with upper gastrointestinal cancers

Disease	Manifestations	Inheritance	Gene(s) detected
Tylosis	Plantar palmar hyperkeratosis Esophageal squamous cell carcinoma	Autosomal dominant Variable pentrance	'TOC' Region 17q25
MEN-1	Multiple parathyroid, pancreatic, pituitary neuroendocrine tumours; upper GI leiomyomas	Autosomal dominant	11q13
Hereditary diffuse gastric cancer	Diffuse gastric cancer Increased risk colon and breast cancer	Autosomal dominant Incomplete penetrance	E-cadherin CDH-1
Familial adenomatous polyposis	Intestinal polyposis (colon>small bowel) Associated with tumours ectodermal origin e.g. epidermoid cysts and desmoid tumours (Gardners) or brain tumours (Turcot syndrome)	Autosomal dominant	APC
Cowden's syndrome	Multiple hamartomas with 40% gastrointestinal polyposis with particular increased risk of colon, thyroid and breast cancer	Autosomal dominant	PTEN Chr 10q
Familial juvenile polyposis	Polyps throughout GI tract, congenital Anomalies (malrotation, hydrocephalus, cardiac lesions) increased risk of colorectal, gastric, duodenal, pancreatic cancer	Autosomal dominant	SMAD4 (DPC4)
Peutz-Jeghers syndrome	Hamartomatous polyps GI tract Mucocutaeous pigmentation GI tumours, pancreatic cancer, genital tumours	Autosomal dominant	STK11 Chr 19p
Neurofibromatosis type 1	Benign and malignant tumours of GI tract	Autosomal dominant	NF1 17q11.2

according to duodenal polyp number, size, histology, and severity of dysplasia (Spigelman *et al.* 1989). A ten-year follow-up study of patients classified using this system demonstrated a significant correlation between the Spigelman stage and the risk of cancer development (56% cancer risk in patients who originally had Spigelman stage 4 disease compared with 2% risk for stage 2 disease) (Groves *et al.* 2002). These data suggest that prophylactic pancreaticoduodenectomy should be considered in patients with advanced but benign duodenal polyposis. Although, it should be remembered that surgery also has associated mortality and morbidity. The alternative treatment is endoscopic polypectomy by means of electrocoagulation and/or laser excision. However, this carries a significant risk of scar formation near the periampullary area and of perforation of the duodenal wall. There is still much progress to be made on surveillance strategies and optimal surgical intervention for these individuals (Koliopanos *et al.* 2002).

For the rare hereditary GI polyposis syndromes such as Besauds–Hillmand–Augier characterised by sexual infantilism, Carter–Horsley–Hughes syndrome, and Ruvalcaba–Myrhe–Smith characterised by dysmorphia and intellectual impairment, it is not clear whether there is an increased risk for malignancy (Haggitt & Reid 1986). They are therefore not included in Table 2.1.

In summary, although progress is being made in identifying the genetic loci for these inherited cancer syndromes, we are only just beginning to face the difficult management decisions that arise from the genetic testing of asymptomatic individuals. For many inherited cancers, no evidence-based preventive measures are yet available and when prevention consists of the removal of target organs, as in the case of HDGC, this is a formidable undertaking. Even when better preventive measures become available, genetic testing will only be appropriate for small populations at high risk under conditions that meet specific criteria.

Low-penetrance genes and upper gastrointestinal cancers

Genetic polymorphisms (variations in genes which account for the normal variability within a population) in low-penetrance genes have been found to increase the cancer risk for many different organ sites. Furthermore, because low-penetrance genetic variants may be common in the population they may account for a substantial fraction of sporadic cancer cases. The prospect of a polygenic approach to common diseases has generated much attention. The question frequently posed is whether or not molecular testing for common variants can have sufficient power to be of practical use either for the individual or for defining risk groups in the population at large.

So far, research efforts have focused mostly on the mechanisms of carcinogen metabolism. For example, genetic variants in the gene cytochrome P450 (CYP) 1A1, which detoxifies the carcinogenic polycyclic aromatic hydrocarbons found in tobacco smoke, may alter the susceptibility to and the survival from lung cancer in Japanese studies (see, for example, Nakachi *et al.* 1991). Recently, a meta-analysis was performed of 50 studies looking at the effect of common alleles of 13 genes on colorectal cancer risk. Polymorphisms in the genes for adenomatosis polyposis (APC), Harvey *ras-1* gene and methylenetetrahydrofolate reductase were found to be the strongest candidates for low-penetrance susceptibility alleles identified to date. However, precise risk estimates will depend on further studies with larger sample sizes (Houlston & Tomlinson 2001). The contribution of low-penetrance susceptibility in oesophageal cancer is not well understood, although progress is being made in gastric cancer. The increasing incidence of oesophageal and gastro-oesophageal junctional tumours in well-defined geographical locations compared with the decline in distal gastric cancer suggests that these diseases have important avoidable environmental determinants. The importance of susceptibility genes therefore has to be understood in the context of the gene-environment interactions.

Low-penetrance susceptibility genes in Barrett's oesophagus

Most patients with reflux symptoms do not develop Barrett's oesophagus (Winters *et al.* 1987; Spechler *et al.* 1994). Furthermore, the degree of reflux exposure and a prior diagnosis of reflux oesophagitis are not accurate predictors for the development of Barrett's oesophagus (Monnier *et al.* 1995; Coenraad *et al.* 1998). This suggests that exposure to gastro-oesophageal reflux is not the sole cause of disease and that there may be a genetic component. However, apart from the rare families with an autosomal pattern of inheritance, it is likely that multiple lower-penetrance genes account for familial clustering of most cases of Barrett's oesophagus.

In a study comparing the relatives of patients with Barrett's oesophagus with their spouse control relatives, the first-degree relatives of Barrett's patients were twice as likely to have heartburn symptoms (Romero *et al.* 1997). A recent study has shown an increased concordance for reflux symptoms in monozygotic pairs, compared with dizygotic pairs. It is estimated that heritability accounted for 31% (23–39%) of the liability to reflux symptoms in this population. (Cameron *et al.* 2002). Unfortunately, whether these individuals with symptoms have pathological evidence of oesophageal disease (oesophagitis or Barrett's oesophagus) and whether they are at an increased risk for developing oesophageal carcinoma is not known.

Low-penetrance susceptibility genes in gastric cancer

Polymorphisms in several candidate genes including *IL1-β*, *IL1-RN*, *CDH1*, *GSTM1*, *GSTP1*, *GSTT1*, *HRAS*, *MTHFR*, *NAT1*, *NAT2*, *TNF-β*, and *TNF-α*, have already been investigated in case–control studies of gastric cancer, but statistically significant associations were only reported for interleukin-1 (*IL-1*: *IL-1β* and *IL1-RN)* (El-Omar *et al.* 2000; Machado *et al.* 2001; Gonzalez *et al.* 2002). However, these studies were conducted using relatively few cases and the statistical power to detect small genetic effects was limited.

Most progress so far has been made with the role of interleukin-1. The importance of *IL-1β* polymorphisms has been confirmed in a Japanese population with a high incidence of gastric cancer (Furuta *et al.* 2002). Furthermore, recent results support the hypothesis that the extent of gastric mucosal injury may be related to *Helicobacter pylori* strain differences, inflammatory responses governed by host genetics, and interactions between host and bacterial determinants (Peek & Blaser 2002). Analysis of the combined bacterial and host genotypes showed that, for each combination, the odds of having gastric carcinoma were greatest in those individuals with both the bacterial and the host high-risk genotypes. Statistical analysis did not reveal any significant interaction between these two groups of factors, suggesting that the risks for developing gastric carcinoma conferred by *H. pylori* and IL-1 genotypes are different. However, the small sample size may have limited the power of the study to detect a small interaction (Blaser 2002; Figueiredo *et al.* 2002). The progress being made in this area demonstrates how assessing risk for upper GI cancers is a tractable problem with the current methodologies available.

Challenge for the future

To detect the low to moderate risks expected to be associated with these and other candidate genetic polymorphisms, much larger case–control series are required. In collaboration with clinicians in East Anglia, we are in the process of setting up a population-based gastric and oesophageal cancer case collection (Stomach Oesophageal Cancer Study, SOCS) with comprehensive epidemiological, clinical and pathological data. This effort has support from the National Translational Cancer Research Network (NTRAC) as part of the National Cancer Research Institute. As a result we have a unique opportunity to collect the many patients required to identify novel genetic and environmental risk factors for these cancers.

Somatic mutations and multi-step concept of carcinogenesis

Motivated by the hope of identifying clinically useful markers for cancer progression, there has been a lot of effort to try to establish the sequence of genetic alterations that occur during the histopathological progression to upper GI cancer. However, it is becoming increasingly clear that although there is an accumulation of abnormalities in oncogenes and tumour suppressor genes in carcinogenesis these pathways may vary between individuals and the sequence of events is not necessarily linear. Furthermore, these studies have been subject to several methodological limitations. Firstly, investigators have usually examined a limited number of somatic mutations at a time, there is variability in the sensitivity and specificity of the different techniques used and the histopathological grading of the degree of dysplasia is undoubtedly variable within and between studies. However, with the advent of microarray technologies, which are able to place a representation of the entire genome on a single slide, there is an opportunity to greatly increase our understanding of the somatic mutations which contribute to cancer development in upper GI cancer tissues and to apply these findings to clinical practice. (For a review of micoarray technology and application to clinical practice, see Aitman (2001).) It is likely that the data generated from these experiments will start to challenge the historical pathological concepts and classifications. Furthermore, many of 'superior' gene expression markers, classifications and prognostic markers will be hypothesised. However, the utility of these approaches will hinge on the bioinformatics available and the validation of the alterations in gene expression that are generated by these techniques.

As well as an understanding of the quantitative changes in gene expression, qualitative changes may also occur (termed cancer epigenetics). For example, promoters of tumour-suppressor genes can be hypermethylated and this methylation status can then be transmitted through cell division. The methyl groups can influence protein–DNA interactions and this may in turn suppress the transcriptional activity of the gene (reviewed by Jones & Laird 1999). New techniques to scan the genome for methylation changes have been developed, and as a result the number of genes known to be affected by methylation in cancer is expanding. This epigenetic silencing of tumour suppressor genes is interesting from a clinical standpoint because it is possible to reverse epigenetic changes and restore function to a cell.

Oesophageal squamous cell carcinoma

Oesophageal squamous cell carcinoma develops as a sequence of histopathological changes that typically involves oesophagitis, atrophy, mild to severe dysplasia, carcinoma *in situ* and eventually invasive cancer over a period of 20 years. The genetic changes associated with the development of oesophageal squamous cell carcinoma include mutation of the p53 gene, disruption of cell cycle control in the G1 phase of the cell cycle, alterations in the retinoblastoma gene RB, activation of oncogenes (*EGFR*, *c-MYC*) and inactivation of several tumour suppressor genes (reviewed in Mandard *et al.* (2000)).

More recently, cDNA microarrays have been used to investigate gene expression profiles in the different stages of oesophageal cancer from the normal squamous oesophagus through to dysplasia and invasive carcinoma. Using a statistical approach called principal component analysis investigators were able to demonstrate that there was a set of genes that were increasingly up or down-regulated in the progression from dysplasia to carcinoma. Furthermore, they were able to idenfity some possible candidate tumour markers (for example a cytokine TNF-α, keratin 6B and S100 calcium binding protein A9), as well as genes involved in cell proliferation and DNA repair (Lu *et al.* 2001). In a study using established oesophageal squamous cell carcinoma cell lines and resection specimens, again multiple cancer-related genes were shown to be differentially expressed. In particular, they were able to show that the oncogene *MET* and its associated protein were overexpressed to a degree that correlated with tumour differentiation (Hu *et al.* 2001). MET encodes a tyrosine kinase receptor for hepatocyte growth factor, and a vast body of clinical and experimental data has demonstrated that MET plays a crucial role in tumourigenesis; however, until now there has been very limited information about its role in squamous oesophageal cancer.

Barrett's oesophagus and oesophageal adenocarcinoma

The progression from Barrett's oesophagus to adenocarcinoma is a multistage process that has been extensively studied to find clinically useful markers for use in surveillance programmes which currently rely on the subjective diagnosis of dysplasia (reviewed in Fitzgerald & Triadafilopoulos (1998); Souza et al. (2001)). Neoplastic progression is associated with alterations in p53, p16 (CDKN2A) and non-random losses of heterozygosity (see Neshat et al. 1994; Barrett et al. 1996; Wong et al. 1997; Maley et al. 2004). In a study examining the evolutionary relationships of these changes it was demonstrated that diploid cell progenitors with somatic or epigenetic (p16 methylation) changes were capable of clonal expansion. The subsequent evolution of neoplastic progeny frequently involved bifurcations and LOH at 5q, 13q and 18q that occurred in no obligate order relative to each other. Hence, the clonal evolution of these tumours appears to be more complex than predicted by linear models.

More recently, it has been demonstrated that cDNA microarrays can differentiate between premalignant Barrett's samples and invasive oesophageal adenocarcinoma. Furthermore, this algorithm could then be used to determine the characteristics of an 'unknown sample' using artificial neural networks. It is hoped that this global gene profiling approach will enable predictions to be made about which patients in the Barrett's population are likely to progress slowly versus quickly (Selaru et al. 2002; Xu et al. 2002) and ultimately to identify specific genes capable of predicting outcome (likelihood for progression).

An alternative approach to cDNA microarrays is to detect loss of heterozygosity and allelic imbalance by using single nucleotide polymorphisms (SNPs). The validity of this approach has been demonstrated in a study in which genome-wide analysis was performed in SNP arrays (600 biallelic markers) on 10 patients with either high-grade dysplasia or oesophageal adenocarcinoma using normal DNA from control gastric tissues (Mei et al. 2000). The SNP array yielded informative loci and it is hoped that with the advent of higher density SNP arrays this will allow efficient, genome-wide high-resolution searches for chromosomal changes associated with tumour initiation and progression which will be able to be used in parallel with cDNA microarray-based methods.

Gastric cancer

Recent molecular analysis of gastric cancer has clarified many genetic alterations in gastric carcinogenesis including p53, β-catenin, E-cadherin, trefoil factor 1 and cmet (reviewed in Yokozaki *et al.* (2001); Hippo *et al.* (2002)). Global gene expression analysis has successfully differentiated cancer from non-cancer tissues as well as identifying genes associated with metastasis (Hippo *et al.* 2002). These results will hopefully pave the way for further studies to provide a new molecular basis for understanding biological properties of gastric cancer. cDNA microarray analysis has also proven to be a useful tool for analysing the complex interplay between *H. pylori* and the host (Maeda *et al.* 2001; Sepulveda *et al.* 2002).

Gene expression profiling and tumour classification

Gene expression profiling has also proven useful in determining upper GI tumour classification and in helping with verification of established cell lines. For example, comparison of gene expression profiling has demonstrated that some cancer cell lines designated as oesophageal adenocarcinomas had an expression profile more similar to that of other squamous cell lines. Furthermore, the gene expression profiles of cancer tissues were remarkably different from those of the cancer cell lines (Kan *et al.* 2001).

One particular classification problem with upper GI malignancies is that of tumours that arise at the gastro-oesophageal junction. It is not clear whether these junctional tumours and tumours of the gastric cardia are genetically similar or distinct from oesophageal adenocarcinomas. From the molecular vantage point, the two cancers share some features, but differ in others (van Dekken *et al.* 1999; El-Rifai *et al.* 2001). For example, *ras* proto-oncogene mutations are rare in both oesophageal and gastric adenocarcinomas and p53 mutations are common in both. Mutations in the adenomatous polyposis coli gene (APC) and microsatellite instability appear to be more important in gastric adenocarcinomas than oesophageal. It is hoped that a global gene expression profile may help to elucidate how these junctional tumours should be classified.

Gene expression profiling as a prognostic and treatment response indicator

Expression profiling is being used to estimate cancer patients' prognosis. For example, a prognostic scoring system for gastric cancer has been developed using a cDNA microarray (Inoue *et al.* 2002). As to the potential for metastases, a global analysis of the differential gene expression of a gastric cancer cell line established from a primary tumour was compared with other cell lines established from the metastasis to the peritoneal cavity (Sakakura *et al.* 2002). This approach enabled the authors to identify several signalling genes that might be important in metastases which had not been reported previously, as well as genes related to cell adhesion and motility, immunity, apoptosis and cell cycle. It is hoped that the identification of such genes might lead to new therapeutic modalities and targets.

In another study, the expression profiles of 20 oesophageal cancer tissues from patients who were treated with the same adjuvant chemotherapy after surgical removal of the tumour were studied in an attempt to find genes associated with the duration of survival after surgery. The authors were able to identify 52 genes that were likely to be correlated with prognosis and possibly with their sensitivity or resistance to the anti-cancer drugs. They also developed a drug response score based on the differential expression of these genes and found a significant correlation between the drug response score and individual patients' prognoses (Kihara *et al.* 2001).

Conclusions

The impact of high-throughput genotyping and gene expression profiling is in its infancy. The challenge will be to interpret the huge amount of data that will be generated from these approaches so as to influence clinical practice for the good. For the minority of the population affected by rare inherited cancer syndromes the challenge is to reduce cancer development once the asymptomatic individuals at risk have been identified. For the commoner sporadic cancer syndromes, the challenge is to use the genetic information to stratify individuals according to their cancer risk and their likely response to specific therapies. Currently, the 5-year survival from upper GI cancers is appalling (less than 10%). These new genetic techniques have the potential to improve the burden of upper GI cancers.

Acknowledgements

We thank Christine Fox for her help with preparation of the manuscript.

References

Aitman, T. J. (2001). DNA microarrays in medical practice. *British Medical Journal* **323**, 6115.

Barrett, M. T., Galipeau, P.C., Sanchez, C. A., Edmond, M. J. & Reid, B. J. (1996). Determination of the frequency of loss of heterozygosity in esophageal adenocarcinoma by cell sorting, whole genome amplification and microsatellite polymorphisms. *Oncogene* **12**, 1873–1878.

Berx, G., Becker, K. F. *et al.* (1998). Mutations of the human E-cadherin (CDH1) gene. *Human Mutation* **12**, 226–237.

Berx, G., Cleton-Jansen, A. M. *et al.* (1995). E-cadherin is a tumour/invasion suppressor gene mutated in human lobular breast cancers. *Embo Journal* **14**, 6107–6115.

Blaser, M. J. (2002). Polymorphic bacteria persisting in polymorphic hosts: assessing *Helicobacter pylori*-related risks for gastric cancer. *Journal of the National Cancer Institute* **94**, 1662–1663.

Cameron, A. J., Lagergren, J. *et al.* (2002). Gastroesophageal reflux disease in monozygotic and dizygotic twins. *Gastroenterology* **122**, 55–59.

Chandrasekharappa, S. C., Guru, S. C. *et al.* (1997). Positional cloning of the gene for multiple endocrine neoplasia-type 1. *Science* **276**, 404–407.

Chun, Y. S., Lindor, N. M. *et al.* (2001). Germline E-cadherin gene mutations: is prophylactic total gastrectomy indicated? *Cancer* **92**, 181–187.

Coenraad, M., Masclee, A. *et al.* (1998). Is Barrett's esophagus characterised by more pronounced acid reflux than severe oesophagitis? *American Journal of Gastroenterology* **93**, 1068–1072.

Dean, P. G., van Heerden, J. A. *et al.* (2000). Are patients with multiple endocrine neoplasia type I prone to premature death? *World Journal of Surgery* **24**, 1437–1441.

Easton, D. & Peto, J. (1990). The contribution of inherited predisposition to cancer incidence. *Cancer Surveys* **9**, 395–416.

Ellis, A., Field, J. K., Field, E. A., Friedmann, P. S., Fryer, A., Howard, P., Leigh, I. M., Risk, J., Shaw, J. M. & Whittaker, J. (1994). Tylosis associated with carcinoma if the oesophagus and oral leukoplakia in a large Liverpool family – a review of six generations. *European Journal of Cancer B Oral Oncology* **30B**, 102–112.

El-Omar, E., Carrington, M. *et al.* (2000). Interleukin-1 polymorphisms associated with increased risk of gastric cancer. *Nature* **404**, 398–402.

El-Rifai, W., Frierson, H. F. Jr, *et al.* (2001). Genetic differences between adenocarcinomas arising in Barrett's esophagus and gastric mucosa. *Gastroenterology* **121**, 592–598.

Figueiredo, C., Machado, J. C. *et al.* (2002). *Helicobacter pylori* and interleukin 1 genotyping: an opportunity to identify high-risk individuals for gastric carcinoma. *Journal of the National Cancer Institute* **94**, 1680–1687.

Fitzgerald, R. & Triadafilopoulos, G. (1998). Recent developments in the molecular characterization of Barrett's esophagus. *Digestive Diseases* **16**, 63–80.

Fitzgerald, R. C. & Caldas, C. (2002). E-cadherin mutations and hereditary gastric cancer: prevention by resection? *Digestive Diseases* **20**, 23–31.

Furuta, T., El-Omar, E. M. *et al.* (2002). Interleukin 1beta polymorphisms increase risk of hypochlorhydria and atrophic gastritis and reduce risk of duodenal ulcer recurrence in Japan. *Gastroenterology* **123**, 92–105.

Gonzalez, C. A., Sala, N. *et al.* (2002). Genetic susceptibility and gastric cancer risk. *International Journal of Cancer* **100**, 249–260.

Grady, W. M., Willis, J. *et al.* (2000). Methylation of the CDH1 promoter as the second genetic hit in hereditary diffuse gastric cancer. *Nature Genetics* **26**, 16–17.

Groves, C. J., Saunders, B. P. *et al.* (2002). Duodenal cancer in patients with familial adenomatous polyposis (FAP): results of a 10 year prospective study. *Gut* **50**, 636–641.

Guilford, P., Hopkins, J. *et al.* (1998). E-cadherin germline mutations in familial gastric cancer. *Nature* **392**, 402–405.

Haggitt, R. C. & Reid, B. J. (1986). Hereditary gastrointestinal polyposis syndromes. *Am Journal of Surgical Pathology* **10**, 871–887.

Hippo, Y., Taniguchi, H. *et al.* (2002). Global gene expression analysis of gastric cancer by oligonucleotide microarrays. *Cancer Research* **62**, 233–240.

Houlston, R. S. & Tomlinson, I. P. (2001). Polymorphisms and colorectal tumor risk. *Gastroenterology* **121**, 282–301.

Hu, Y. C., Lam, K. Y. *et al.* (2001). Profiling of differentially expressed cancer-related genes in esophageal squamous cell carcinoma (ESCC) using human cancer cDNA arrays: overexpression of oncogene MET correlates with tumor differentiation in ESCC. *Clinical Cancer Research* **7**, 3519–3525.

Huntsman, D. G., Carneiro, F. *et al.* (2001). Early gastric cancer in young, asymptomatic carriers of germ-line E-cadherin mutations. *New England Journal of Medicine* **344**, 1904–1909.

Inoue, H., Matsuyama, A. *et al.* (2002). Prognostic score of gastric cancer determined by cDNA microarray. *Clinical Cancer Research* **8**, 3475–3479.

Jones, P. A. & Laird, P. W. (1999). Cancer epigenetics comes of age. *Nature Genetics* **21**, 163–167.

Kan, T., Shimada, Y. *et al.* (2001). Gene expression profiling in human esophageal cancers using cDNA microarray. *Biochemical and Biophysical Research Communications* **286**, 792–801.

Keller, G., Vogelsang, H. *et al.* (1999). Diffuse type gastric and lobular breast carcinoma in a familial gastric cancer patient with an E-cadherin germline mutation. *American Journal of Pathology* **155**, 337–342.

Kihara, C., Tsunoda, T. *et al.* (2001). Prediction of sensitivity of esophageal tumors to adjuvant chemotherapy by cDNA microarray analysis of gene-expression profiles. *Cancer Research* **61**, 6474–6479.

Knudson, A. G. Jr (1985). Hereditary cancer, oncogenes, and anti-oncogenes. *Cancer Research* **45**, 1437–1443.

Koliopanos, A., Wirtz, M. *et al.* (2002). The role of surgery in the prevention of familial cancer syndromes of the gastrointestinal tract. *Digestive Diseases* **20**, 91–101.

Larsson, C., Skogseid, B. *et al.* (1988). Multiple endocrine neoplasia type 1 gene maps to chromosome 11 and is lost in insulinoma. *Nature* **332**, 85–87.

Lu, J., Liu, Z. *et al.* (2001). Gene expression profile changes in initiation and progression of squamous cell carcinoma of esophagus. *International Journal of Cancer* **91**, 288–294.

Machado, J. C., Oliveira, C. *et al.* (2001). E-cadherin gene (CDH1) promoter methylation as the second hit in sporadic diffuse gastric carcinoma. *Oncogene* **20**, 1525–1528.

Maeda, S., Otsuka, M. *et al.* (2001). cDNA microarray analysis of *Helicobacter pylori*-mediated alteration of gene expression in gastric cancer cells. *Biochemical and Biophysical Research Communications* **284**, 443–449.

Maley, C. C., Galipeau, P. C., Li, X., Sanchez, C. A., Paulson, T. G. & Reid, B. J. (2004). Selectively advantageous mutations and hitchhikers in neoplasms: p16 lesions are selected in Barrett's esophagus. *Cancer Research,* **64**, 3414–3427.

Mandard, A. M., Hainaut, P. *et al.* (2000). Genetic steps in the development of squamous cell carcinoma of the esophagus. *Mutation Research* **462**, 335–342.

McKeeby, J. L., Li, X. *et al.* (2001). Multiple leiomyomas of the esophagus, lung, and uterus in multiple endocrine neoplasia type 1. *American Journal of Pathology* **159**, 1121–1127.

Mei, R., Galipeau, P. C. *et al.* (2000). Genome-wide detection of allelic imbalance using human SNPs and high-density DNA arrays. *Genome Research* **10**, 1126–1137.

Monnier, P., Ollyo, J.-P. *et al.* (1995). Epidemiology and natural history of reflux esophagitis. *Seminars in Laparoscopic Surgery* **2**, 2–9.

Nakachi, K., Imai, K. *et al.* (1991). Genetic susceptibility to squamous cell carcinoma of the lung in relation to cigarette smoking dose. *Cancer Research* **51**, 5177–5180.

Neshat, K., Sanchez, C. A., Galipeau, P. C., Cowan, D. S., Ramel, S., Levine, D. S. & Reid, B. J. (1994). P53 mutations in Barrett's adenocarcinoma and high-grade dysplasia. *Gastroenterology* **106**, 1589–1595.

Nugent, K. P., Spigelman, A. D. *et al.* (1993). Life expectancy after colectomy and ileorectal anastomosis for familial adenomatous polyposis. *Diseases of the Colon and Rectum* **36**, 1059–1062.

Peek, R. M. Jr & Blaser, M. J. (2002). *Helicobacter pylori* and gastrointestinal tract adenocarcinomas. *Nature Reviews Cancer* **2**, 28–37.

Pharoah, P. D., Guildford, P. & Caldas, C. (2001). Incidence of gastric cancer and breast cancer in CDH1 (E-cadherin) mutation carriers from hereditary diffuse gastric cancer families. *Gastroenterology* **121**, 1348–1353.

Richards, F. M., McKee, S. A. *et al.* (1999). Germline E-cadherin gene (CDH1) mutations predispose to familial gastric cancer and colorectal cancer. *Human Molecular Genetics* **8**, 607–610.

Risk, J. M., Evans, K. E. *et al.* (2002). Characterization of a 500 kb region on 17q25 and the exclusion of candidate genes as the familial tylosis oesophageal cancer (TOC) locus. *Oncogene* **21**, 6395–6402.

Risk, J. M., Mills, H. S. *et al.* (1999). The tylosis esophageal cancer (TOC) locus: more than just a familial cancer gene. *Diseases of the Esophagus* **12**, 173–176.

Romero, Y., Cameron, A. *et al.* (1997). Familial aggregation of gastroesophageal reflux in patients with Barrett's esophagus and esophageal adenocarcinoma. *Gastroenterology* **113**, 1449–1456.

Romero, Y. and Locke, G. R. III (1999). Is there a GERD gene? *American Journal of Gastroenterology* **94**, 1127–1129.

Sakakura, C., Hagiwara, A. *et al.* (2002). Differential gene expression profiles of gastric cancer cells established from primary tumour and malignant ascites. *British Journal of Cancer* **87**, 1153–1161.

Selaru, F. M., Zou, T., Xu, Y., Shustova, V., Yin, J., Mori, Y., Sato, F., Wang, S., Olaru, A., Shibata, D., Greenwald, E. D., Krasna, M. J., Abraham, J. M. & Meltzer, S. J. (2002). Global gene expression profiling in Barrett's esophagus and esophageal cancer: a comparative analysis using cDNA microarrays. *Oncogene* **21**, 475–478.

Sepulveda, A. R., Tao, H. *et al.* (2002). Screening of gene expression profiles in gastric epithelial cells induced by *Helicobacter pylori* using microarray analysis. *Alimentary Pharmacology and Therapeutics* 16 (Suppl. 2), 145–157.

Skogseid, B., Oberg, K. *et al.* (1996). Surgery for asymptomatic pancreatic lesion in multiple endocrine neoplasia type I. *World Journal of Surgery* **20**, 872–876; discussion 877.

Souza, R. F., Morales, C. P. *et al.* (2001). A conceptual approach to understanding the molecular mechanisms of cancer development in Barrett's oesophagus. *Alimentary Pharmacology and Therapeutics* **15**, 1087–1100.

Spechler, S. J., Zeroogian, J. M. *et al.* (1994). Prevalence of metaplasia at the gastro-esophageal junction. *The Lancet* **344**, 1533–1536.

Spigelman, A. D., Williams, C. B. *et al.* (1989). Upper gastrointestinal cancer in patients with familial adenomatous polyposis. *The Lancet* **2**, 783–785.

Thompson, N. W. (1998). Current concepts in the surgical management of multiple endocrine neoplasia type 1 pancreatic-duodenal disease. Results in the treatment of 40 patients with Zollinger-Ellison syndrome, hypoglycaemia or both. *Journal of Internal Medicine* **243**, 495–500.

Van Dekken, H., Geelen, E. *et al.* (1999). Comparative genomic hybridization of cancer of the gastroesophageal junction: deletion of 14Q31-32.1 discriminates between esophageal (Barrett's) and gastric cardia adenocarcinomas. *Cancer Research* **59**, 748–752.

Winters, C., Spurling, T. *et al.* (1987). Barrett's esophagus: a prevalent occult complication of gastro-oesophageal reflux disease. *Gastroenterology* **92**, 118–124.

Wong, D. J., Barrett, M. T., Stoger, R., Emond, M. J. & Reid, B. J. (1997). P16NK4a promoter is hypermethylated at high frequency in esophageal adenocarcinoma. *Cancer Research* **57**, 2619–2622.

Xu, Y., Selaru, F. M., Yin, J., Zou, T. T., Shustova, V., Mori, Y., Sato, F., Liu, T. C., Olaru, A., Wang, S., Kimos, M. C., Perry, K., Desai, K., Greenwald, B. D., Krasna, M. J., Shibata, D., Abraham, J. M. & Meltzer, S. J. (2002). Artificial neural networks and gene filtering distinguish between global gene expression profiles of Barrett's esophagus and esophageal cancer. *Cancer Research* **62**, 3493–3497.

Yokozaki, H., Yasui, W. *et al.* (2001). Genetic and epigenetic changes in stomach cancer. *International Review of Cytology* **204**, 49–95.

Chapter 3

Intervention and surveillance strategies for Barrett's oesophagus

Janusz A Jankowski, Stephen Attwood, Hugh Barr, Paul Moayyedi and Peter Watson

Oesophagitis secondary to gastro-oesophageal reflux disease (GORD) is arguably the most common medical condition in Western countries, with 30% of adults complaining of heartburn at least once per month (Jankowski *et al.* 2000a; Spechler *et al.* 2001). Ten per cent of patients with oesophagitis will progress to Barrett's metaplasia (BM), which is a premalignant mucin-secreting columnar epithelium that lines the distal oesophagus (Jankowski *et al.* 2000; Schnell *et al.* 2001). Whereas dysplasia in BM is still the gold standard for assessing the premalignant potential, most individuals present with their adenocarcinoma. Furthermore, even 'high-grade dysplasia' has recently been shown to be an unreliable marker of cancer risk in a 5 year period (Schnell *et al.* 2001; Spechler *et al.* 2001). In addition, the diagnosis of dysplasia in BM usually occurs when an individual is already under endoscopic follow-up in a surveillance programme, which clearly has additional economic implications that have not as yet been shown to be cost effective. Consequently, it is the commonly diagnosed BM at which intervention needs to be assessed. However, the rationale for medical intervention before dysplasia or indeed neoplasia develops currently lacks a satisfactory evidence base. In this, the UK has one of the highest worldwide prevalences of BM: 0.5–2% of adults have BM resulting in an incidence of oesophageal adenocarcinoma, which is three to four times that seen in either Europe or North America (Jankowski *et al.* 2000b). In addition, the conversion rate to cancer of individuals with BM in surveillance programmes is twice as common in the UK compared with the USA, lending further support to the notion that the UK is a high-risk region. This is interesting especially because genetic factors may occasionally play a role in a small proportion of BM, as this lesion can have familial clustering and occurs in twins (Jankowski *et al.* 2002). The incidence of BM neoplastic change each year in the UK is between 0.76% and 1.2%. The resulting adenocarcinoma is characterised by a uniformly poor prognosis: a median survival time, after diagnosis, of less than 1 year, and fewer than 10% of patients surviving for more than 5 years despite modern combined chemotherapy and surgery. Hence, the ideal requirement is to detect lesions at an earlier stage where intervention has dramatically improved survival benefits (Sarr *et al.* 1985). The conventional clinical risk factors for the development of Barrett's adenocarcinoma have not yet been proven in a randomised controlled study (Skinner *et al.* 1983; Spechler *et al.* 1983; Cameron *et al.* 1992; Gray *et al.* 1993; Menke-Pluymers *et al.* 1993; Morgan *et al.* 1998; Morales *et al.* 1999; Lagergren *et al.* 1999a,b, 2000; Weston *et al.* 2000). Therefore, in the absence of proven stratification, surveillance of all cases of Barrett's metaplasia is required, which currently is neither feasible nor cost effective (Jankowski *et al.* 1999). Consequently, attention has centred on a greater understanding of the basic biology so that novel therapeutic strategies can be identified early in progression. Specifically, interest has been rekindled in primary prevention strategies aimed at reducing the initiation of BM and detecting additional risk factors, which more accurately predict the subgroups that will progress to malignancy. These include intermediate markers such as aneuploidy, p16 p53 mutations, cyclin D1 expression and altered catenin biology (Malescic *et al.* 1996). Many interventions have been tried to prevent the progression of BM to cancer, but it is the pharmaceutical manipulation of the oesophagus that which have the greatest applicability. 'Mass cancer prevention requires mass interventions' (*vide infra*).

Gastro-oesophageal reflux of acid and bile are the predominant initiating factors in Barrett's metaplasia, although the precise mechanism of cytotoxicity is unclear. Proton pump inhibitors (PPIs) are widely used in the treatment of Barrett's metaplasia, as in 2002 this indication alone accounted for a cost of £60 million to the NHS. They are highly effective and safe in minimising symptoms and healing of squamous oesophagitis, but there is no clear evidence that they inhibit the evolution of preneoplastic BM. One of the main problems is that there are no antecedent clinical studies that have addressed this issue. However, proof of concept for the notion that PPIs can reduce cancer risk comes from observations that partial regression of metaplastic mucosa may be induced by suppression of acid (and bile) reflux with either PPIs or anti-reflux surgery (McDonald *et al.* 1996; Peters *et al.* 1999). Furthermore, in the latter group of patients with successful anti-reflux surgery, subsequent neoplastic change decreased over subsequent follow-up over periods between 5 and 15 years. In the shorter term, intermediate markers on metaplastic biopsies from patients with Barrett's metaplasia in whom intraoesophageal pH had been normalised on PPI therapy showed decreased cell proliferation and improved differentiation. Alternatively, incomplete acid suppression that allows short pulses of acid led to epithelial changes, which could be interpreted as selecting poorly differentiated cells with increased proliferative potential (Triadafilopoulos 2000). These latter authors have concluded that the population of patients with BM represents a heterogeneous group with a variable response to proton pump inhibition despite apparent symptom control. Taken together, these data indicate that gastro-oesophageal reflux is implicated in the pathogenesis of BM; there is preliminary evidence to show that its attenuation reverses the surrogate markers in the short term, the metaplastic histology in the medium term, and the cancer risk in the longer term.

There is a counter-argument that PPIs may not be protective against oesophageal cancer. Evidence from epidemiological studies suggests that since the widespread introduction of potent acid-suppressing drugs (H2 antagonists and PPIs), oesophageal adenocarcinoma has increased dramatically (Sharma *et al.* 2004). Furthermore, in animal models of duodenogastric reflux, there is an enhanced cancer risk especially when gastric acid blockade by omeprazole is used (Wetscher *et al.* 1999; Van Laethem *et al.* 2000). Bile acids may be physiologically more cytotoxic at a neutral pH, and it is therefore theoretically possible that PPI therapy could promote oesophageal cancer in humans. This is perhaps offset by a reduction in bile reflux in patients on PPIs, as measured by bilitec monitoring (Van Laethem *et al.* 2000). On the basis of these observations, it is likely that any cytotoxic modifying effects of PPIs, either directly or indirectly, are determined by the extent and/or pattern of acid suppression. Because Barrett's mucosa is relatively insensitive to acid (Katzka & Castell 1994; Murphy *et al.* 1994; Ortiz *et al.* 1999), symptom control is easier to achieve than normalisation of intra-oesophageal pH (Ouatu-Lascar *et al.* 1998; Castell *et al.* 2001). Symptoms are, however, an unreliable guide to the degree of acid reflux and cannot be relied on as a guide to the adequacy of treatment. Most patients' reflux symptoms are controlled with a once-daily standard dose of PPI, but normalisation of intra-oesophageal pH is achieved in fewer than 50% (Edwards *et al.* 2001). Normalisation of pH can usually be achieved with twice-daily dosage of PPI, but some patients require even higher doses although recent evidence indicates that esomeprazole (Nexium) is more effective than other PPIs in more severe reflux disease (Edwards *et al.* 2001).

Another major issue is why the metaplasia does not regress once the external stimulus for its initiation is removed. Some evidence suggests that COX-2 may be one of the molecules responsible because it is expressed constitutively in metaplastic but not normal or inflamed squamous oesophageal mucosa. Non-selective COX-2 inhibitors such as aspirin and non-steroidal anti-inflammatory drugs (NSAIDs) have been shown to be associated with a decreased incidence of oesophageal and gastric adenocarcinoma, as well as for the colorectum (Sharma *et al.* 2004). However, non-selective NSAIDs including aspirin have a side-effect profile such as upper gastrointestinal ulceration and risk of gastrointestinal haemorrhage, which is a relative contraindication to their use. COX-2 is implicated in cellular adaptation in epithelia in injured or inflamed mucosa, and its expression is increased serially along the metaplasia–dysplasia–adenocarcinoma sequence, especially in advanced Barrett's cancer (Shirvani *et al.* 2000; Morris *et al.* 2001). Furthermore, the up-regulation of COX-2 expression is at a very early stage in low-grade dysplasia, with all cases of high-grade dysplasia having a several-fold increased COX-2 compared with benign Barrett's metaplasia (Shirvani *et al.* 2000). We have also recently shown that COX-2 inhibitors can suppress levels of this protein in both untransfected and maximally expressing COX-2 oesophageal cells. Selection of COX-2 inhibition may be an important chemoprevention strategy in oesophageal cancer alone, regardless of acid reflux levels (Souza *et al.* 2000; Li *et al.* 2000), and rofecoxib (50 mg/day) suppresses more than 95% of prostaglandin synthesis in the mucosa with minimal side effects.

At present, the cost of resection of oesophageal adenocarcinoma is £12,000 per patient. Despite this, the success is at best dismal, with a 20% 5-year survival and frequent life-threatening complications. Intervention at earlier stages when dysplasia is present is not much better, with treatment costing £1,000 per course of mucosal ablation therapy and life-threatening complications are relatively common; even then there is no guarantee of cancer prevention. In this regard, we believe that pharmaceutical chemoprevention of Barrett's adenocarcinoma is the best intervention. The cost of intervention with full symptomatic doses of PPIs and COX-2 inhibitor therapy is £400 annually, and complications are infrequent and usually self-limiting.

As mentioned previously, there are unfortunately no randomised controlled trials addressing the issue of surveillance of Barrett's metaplasia. We do, however, have access to over 40 single-centre reports detailing the cancer conversion rate. In many reports it has been recognised that there is a publication bias to more extreme results; however, in UK studies this is not the case. In the UK, when allowing for publication bias and prevalence of cancers (diagnosed in the first year of surveillance), the annual incidence of oesophageal adenocarcinoma is 0.98% compared with 0.5% in North America. There seems little argument that those cancers diagnosed in a surveillance program tend to be at a much earlier stage of development and usually have a better prognosis. However, at least 25% of patients with these early cancers will not be able to undergo surgery because of shared co-morbidities such as ischaemic heart disease and cerebrovascular or peripheral vascular disease. Therefore, most cancers are not picked up in surveillance programmes, and those that are may not always benefit from surgical intervention.

In conclusion, several strategies are available for intervention in those at risk from Barrett's adenocarcinoma. Most notably, these are surveillance endoscopy and ablation therapies and chemoprevention; however, no data are available to justify either approach. There is a great need for randomised controlled trials assessing these issues in the immediate future.

References

Cameron, A. J. & Lomboy, C. T. 91992). Barrett's esophagus: age, prevalence and extent of columnar epithelium. *Gastroenterology* **103**, 1241–1245.

Castell, D. O., Kahrilas, P. J., Richter, J. E., Vakil, N. B., Johnson, D. A., Zuckerman, S., Skammer, W. & Levine, J. G. (2002). Esomeprazole (40 mg) compared with lansoprazole (30 mg) in the treatment of erosive esophagitis. *American Journal of Gastroenterology* **97**, 575–583.

Edwards, S. J., Lind, T. & Lundell, L. (2001). Systematic review of proton pump inhibitors for the acute treatment of reflux oesophagitis. *Alimentary Pharmacology and Therapeutics* **15**, 1729–1736.

Gray, M. R., Donnelly, R. J. & Kingsnorth, A. N. (1993). The role of smoking and alcohol in metaplasia and cancer risk in Barrett's oesophagus. *Gut* **34**, 727–731.

Jankowski, J., Wright, N. A., Meltzer, S., Triadafilopoulos, G., Geboes, K., Casson, A., Kerr, D. & Young, L. S. (1999). Molecular evolution of the metaplasia dysplasia adenocarcinoma sequence in the esophagus (MCS). *American Journal of Pathology* **154**, 965–974.

Jankowski, J., Harrison, R.F., Perry, I., Balkwill, F. & Tselepis, C. (2000). Seminar: Barrett's metaplasia. *The Lancet* **356**, 2079–2085.

Jankowski, J., Perry, I. & Harrison, R. F. (2000). Gastro-oesophageal cancer: death at the junction. *British Medical Journal* **321**, 463–464.

Jankowski, J., Provenzale, D. & Moayyedi, P. (2002). Oesophageal adenocarcinoma arising from Barrett's metaplasia has regional variations in the West. *Gastroenterology* **122**, 588–590.

Katzka, D. A. & Castell, D. O. (1994). Successful elimination of reflux symptoms does not ensure adequate control of acid reflux in patients with Barrett's esophagus. *American Journal of Gastroenterology* **89**, 989–991.

Lagergren, J., Bergstrom, R., Lindgren, A. G. & Nyren, O. (1999). Symptomatic gastroesophageal reflux as a risk factor for esophageal adenocarcinoma. *New England Journal of Medicine* **340**, 825–831.

Lagergren, J., Berstrom, R. & Nyren, O. (1999). Association between body mass and adenocarcinoma of the esophagus. *Annals of Internal Medicine* **130**, 883–890.

Lagergren, J., Bergstrom, R., Adami, H. O. & Nyren, O. (2000). Association between medications that relax the lower esophageal sphincter and risk for esophageal adenocarcinoma. *Annals of Internal Medicine* **133**, 165–175.

Malesci, A., Savarino, V., Zentilin, P., Belicchi, M., Mela, G. S., Lapertosa, G., Bocchia, P., Ronchi, G. & Franceschi, M. (1996). Partial regression of Barrett's esophagus by long-term therapy with high-dose omeprazole. *Gastrointestinal Endoscopy* **44**, 700–705.

McDonald, M. L., Trastek, V. F., Allen, M. S., Deschamps, C. & Pairolero, P. C. (1996). Barrett's esophagus: does an antireflux procedure reduce the need for endoscopic surveillance? *Journal of Thoracic and Cardiovascular Surgery* **111**, 1135–1138.

Menke-Pluymers, M. B. E., Hop, W. C. J., Dees, J., van Blankenstein, M. & Tilanus, H. W. (1993). Risk factors for the development of an adenocarcinoma in Barrett's oesophagus. *Cancer* **72**, 1155–1158.

Morales, T. G. & Sampliner, R. E. (1999). Barrett's esophagus: an update on screening, surveillance and treatment. *Archives of Internal Medicine* **159**, 1411–1416.

Morgan, G. & Vainio, H. (1998). Barrett's oesophagus, oesophageal cancer and colon cancer: an explanation of the association and cancer chemopreventative potential of non-steroidal anti-inflammatory drugs. *European Journal of Cancer Prevention* **7**, 195–199.

Morris, C. D., Armstrong, G. R., Bigley, G., Green, H. & Attwood, S. E. (2001). Cyclooxygenase-2 expression in the Barrett's metaplasia–dysplasia–adenocarcinoma sequence. *American Journal of Gastroenterology* **96**, 990–906.

Ortiz, A., Martinez de Haro, L. F., Parrilla, P., Molina, J., Bermejo, J. & Munitiz, V. (1999). 24-hour pH monitoring is necessary to assess acid reflux suppression in patients with Barrett's oesophagus undergoing treatment with proton pump inhibitors. *British Journal of Surgery* **86**, 1472–1474.

Ouatu-Lascar, R. & Triadafilopoulos, G. (1998). Complete elimination of reflux symptoms does not guarantee normalization of intraesophageal acid reflux in patients with Barrett's esophagus. *American Journal of Gastroenterology* **93**, 711–716.

Peters, F. T., Ganesh, S., Kuipers, E. J., Sluiter, W. J., Klinkenberg-Knol, E. C., Lamers, C. B. & Kleibeuker, J. H. (1999). Endoscopic regression of Barrett's oesophagus during omeprazole treatment; a randomized double blind study. *Gut* **45**, 489–494.

Romero, Y., Cameron, A. J., Locke, G. R., Schaid, D. J., Slezak, J. M., Breanch, C. D. & Melton, L. J. (1997). Familial aggregation of gastroesophageal reflux in patients with Barrett's esophagus and esophageal adenocarcinoma. *Gastroenterology* **113**, 1449–1456.

Sarr, M. G., Hamilton, S. R., Marrone, G. C. & Cameron, J. L. (1985). Barrett's esophagus: its prevalence and association with adenocarcinoma in patients with symptoms of gastroesophageal reflux. *American Journal of Surgery* **149**, 187–193.

Schnell, T. G., Sontag, S., Chejfec, G., Aranha, G., Metz, A., O'Connell, S., Seidel, U. & Sonnenberg, A. (2001). Long-term nonsurgical management of Barrett's esophagus with high-grade dysplasia. *Gastroenterology* **120**, 1607–1619.

Sharma, P., McQuaid, K., Dent, J., Fennerty, M. B., Sampliner, R., Spechler, S. J., Cameron, A., Corley, D., Falk, G., Goldblum, J. *et al.* (2004). A critical review of the diagnosis and management of Barrett's esophagus: the AGA Chicago Workshop. *Gastroenterology* **127**, 310–330.

Shirvani, V. N., Quatu-Lascar, R., Kaur, B. S., Omary, M. B. & Triadafilopoulos, G. (2000). Cyclooxygenase-2 expression in Barrett's esophagus and adenocarcinoma: ex vivo induction by bile salts and acid exposure. *Gastroenterology* **118**, 487–496.

Skinner, D. B., Walther, B. C., Riddell, R. H., Schmidt, H., Iascone, C. & DeMeester, T. (1983). Barrett's esophagus. *Annals of Surgery* **198**, 554–566.

Souza, R. F., Shewmake, K., Beer, D. G., Cryer, B. & Spechler, S. J. (2000). Selective inhibition of cyclooxygenase-2 suppresses growth and induces apoptosis in human esophageal adenocarcinoma cells. *Cancer Research* **60**, 5767–5772.

Spechler, S. J., Sperber, H., Doos, W. G. & Schimmel, E. M. (1983). The prevalence of Barrett's esophagus in patients with chronic peptic esophageal strictures. *Digestive Diseases and Sciences* **28**, 769–774.

Spechler, S. J., Lee, E., Ahnen, D., Goyal, R. K., Hirano, I., Ramirez, F., Raufman, J. P., Sampliner, R., Schnell, T., Sontag, S., Vlahcevic, Z. R., Young, R. & Williford, W. (2001). Long-term outcome of medical and surgical therapies for gastroesophageal reflux disease. *Journal of the American Medical Association* **285**, 2376–2378.

Triadafilopoulos, G. (2000). Proton pump inhibitors for Barrett's oesophagus. *Gut* **46**, 144–146.

Van Laethem, J. L., Peny, M. O., Salmon, I., Cremer, M. & Deviere, J. (2000). Intramucosal adenocarcinoma arising under squamous re-epithelialisation of Barrett's oesophagus. *Gut* **46**, 574–547.

Weston, A. P., Badr, A. S., Topalovski, M., Cherian, R., Dixon, A. & Hassanein, R. S. (2000). Propective evaluation of the prevalence of gastric Helicobacter pylori infection in patients with GERD, Barrett's esophagus, Barrett's dysplasia, and Barrett's adenocarcinoma. *American Journal of Gastroenterology* **95**, 387–394.

Wetscher, G. J., Hinder, R. A., Smyrk, T., Perdikis, G., Adrian, T. E. & Profanter, C. (1999). Gastric acid blockade with omeprazole promotes gastric carcinogenesis induced by duodenogastric reflux. *Digestive Diseases and Sciences* **44**, 1132–1135.

PART 2

Gastro-oesophageal cancer

Chapter 4

Peri-operative chemotherapy in oesophago-gastric cancer

James Dickson, Sheela Rao, Ian Chau and David Cunningham

Introduction

Oesophago-gastric cancer is the second most common cancer in the world and the one of the most frequent causes of cancer-related mortality. Oesophageal cancer accounts for approximately 400,000 new cases and 340,000 cancer-related deaths worldwide (Ferlay *et al.* 2001). In the UK this represents approximately 7,000 new cases and 6,800 deaths per year. In addition, gastric cancer, although declining in incidence, is the eighth most common cause of cancer-related mortality. It accounts for approximately 875,000 new cases and 645,000 deaths worldwide, with approximately 10,000 new cases, with 8,300 deaths per year in the UK (Ferlay *et al.* 2001). The epidemiology of oesophago-gastric cancer, in Western countries, is changing with a significant increase in the incidence of adenocarcinoma of the lower oesophagus, oesophago-gastric junction and cardia of the stomach for both sexes (Vizcaino *et al.* 2002). In contrast, the incidence of gastric cancer, in particular tumours of the fundus and antrum of the stomach, is decreasing.

Prognostic factors for patients who undergo resection include the type of resection (R), depth of invasion (T), the presence and number of nodal metastases (N), and the ratio of involved to removed lymph nodes. In addition to these clinico-pathological factors, molecular markers have also been shown to be of prognostic value. In oesophageal adenocarcinoma arising in Barrett's oesophagus, p53 mutations correlated with inferior survival (Schneider *et al.* 2000). Furthermore, in squamous cell carcinoma of the oesophagus, p53 mutations have been associated with decreased sensitivity to radiotherapy (Miyata *et al.* 2000), and VEGF expression with nodal metastases and poorer survival (Shih *et al.* 2000). For gastric carcinoma, expression of Her-2/neu (Allgayer *et al.* 2000), TGF-ß and EGFR (Kuwahara *et al.* 1999), and PDGR-A (Katano *et al.* 1998) have been associated with poorer survival. In addition, high expression of thymidylate synthase and excision repair cross complementary (ERCC)-1 gene are associated with poor prognosis in patients receiving platinum- and fluoropyrimidine-based chemotherapy (Metzger *et al.* 1998). The prognosis of oesophago-gastric cancer is poor, with a 5-year survival of only 5–10% for oesophageal cancer and 10–20% for gastric cancer (Table 4.1). This is due to most (70–80%) patients having locally advanced or metastatic disease before symptoms occur, with early spread, and close anatomic proximity to vital organs, making treatment difficult. Hence, only 20–30% of patients are potentially curable with surgery alone.

Table 4.1 Five-year survival rates for oesophago-gastric cancer

	England and Wales	Europe	USA
Oesophageal cancer	6%	8%	13.7%
Gastric cancer	10%	20%	21.8%

The rationale for administering neoadjuvant chemotherapy is to achieve tumour downstaging to improve the curative resection (R0) rate, and to eliminate micrometastatic disease to improve disease-free and overall survival. In addition, adjuvant chemotherapy is generally poorly tolerated following surgery in this group of patients. Furthermore, pathological evaluation of response to therapy also adds prognostic information.

Surgery is considered the treatment of choice for most patients with localised oesophago-gastric cancer; the objective being the achievement of a curative resection (R0), that constitutes the removal of all gross tumour and regional lymph nodes, with clear resection margins. However, those patients who have undergone a curative resection and who represent the best prognostic group have a median survival of 25 months, and a 5-year survival rate of only 20–30%. Based on the poor survival figures, there is clearly room for improvement.

Neoadjuvant chemotherapy in oesophageal cancer

Two large randomised studies evaluating the role of neoadjuvant chemotherapy in localised oesophageal cancer have recently been published. The United Kingdom Medical Research Council (MRC) OEO2, reported by the MRC Oesophageal Cancer Working Party (2000), is the largest study to address this issue. A total of 802 previously untreated patients were randomly allocated to either two 4-day cycles of cisplatin (80 mg/m^2 on day 1) and 5-fluorouracil (1,000 mg/m^2 by protracted venous infusion (PVI) on days 1–4) every three weeks followed by surgical resection or surgery alone. Overall survival was better in the neoadjuvant chemotherapy arm (hazard ratio (HR) 0.79; 95% confidence interval (CI) 0.67–0.93; $p = 0.004$) compared with surgery alone. Two-year survival rates were 43% in the neoadjuvant chemotherapy arm versus 34% in the surgery alone arm. Disease-free survival was also better in the neoadjuvant chemotherapy arm (HR 0.75; 95% CI 0.63–0.89; $p = 0.0014$).

The second-largest study addressing this issue was the Intergroup 113 study (Kelsen *et al.* 1998), conducted in the USA. A total of 440 previously untreated patients were randomly assigned to either three 5-day cycles of cisplatin (100 mg/m^2 on day 1) and 5-fluorouracil (1,000 mg/m^2 /day by PVI on days 1–5) every four weeks followed by surgical resection or surgery alone. Post-operative chemotherapy with a reduced dose of cisplatin was advocated in patients with stable or responsive disease. There was no difference in overall survival between the two arms (HR 1.07; 95% CI 0.87 to 1.32; p = 0.53). Two-year survival rates were 35% in the neoadjuvant chemotherapy arm versus 37% in the surgery alone arm. There was no significant difference in disease-free survival between the two groups (p = 0.50).The conflicting results from these two studies warrant further discussion. A comparison between the MRC and Intergroup studies is shown in Table 4.2. The results cannot be explained by differences in the baseline characteristics of the study populations, which were similar. However, although both cisplatin and 5-fluorouracil were used in the neoadjuvant chemotherapy arm of both trials, the Intergroup study used a higher dose of cisplatin for three cycles, versus two cycles in the MRC study, and in addition also gave adjuvant chemotherapy. The two year survival rates were similar in the surgery alone arms (34% versus 37%), so it may be possible that the toxicity associated with the higher total dose of neoadjuvant chemotherapy in the Intergroup study (cisplatin 300 mg/m^2 and 5-fluorouracil 15,000 mg/m^2 over 8 weeks versus cisplatin 160 mg/m^2 and 5-fluorouracil 8,000 mg/m^2 over 3 weeks) nullified any potential survival benefit, as seen in the MRC study. This is illustrated by the fact that only 71% of patients completed their course of neoadjuvant chemotherapy, versus 90% in the MRC study. Furthermore, only 80% of patients in the neoadjuvant chemotherapy arm of the Intergroup study proceeded to surgery, compared with 92% in the MRC study.

Table 4.2 Comparison of the MRC OEO2 and Intergroup 113 studies

	Surgery	Chemotherapy + Surgery	Surgery	Chemotherapy + Surgery
Number of patients	402	400	227	213
Histology				
Squamous	31%	31%	47%	46%
Adenocarcinoma	67%	66%	53%	54%
Surgery performed				
Yes	97%	92%	96%	80%
No	3%	8%	4%	20%
R0 resection	54%	60%	59%	62%
Pathological CR rate	NA	4%	NA	2.5%
Median survival (months)	13.3	16.8	16.1	14.9
2-year survival	34%	43%	37%	35%

CR, complete response; NA, not applicable; R0, microscopic complete resection.

In addition, for those patients in the neoadjuvant chemotherapy arms of the two studies, the median delay to surgery was 63 days in the MRC study, versus 93 days in the Intergroup study. This longer delay before surgery is potentially significant, particularly in the group of patients who do not respond to neoadjuvant chemotherapy. These clinical non-responders have worse survival than those who proceed to immediate surgery, and this may contribute to the overall neutral impact of neoadjuvant chemotherapy on overall and disease-free survival in the Intergroup study. Interestingly, in the Intergroup study, patients who responded to neoadjuvant chemotherapy had a significantly better survival rate than non-responders ($p = 0.002$) and those in the surgery alone arm ($p < 0.001$) (Kelsen et al. 1999). For surgery performed, the proportion of microscopically complete resections (R0) achieved in both studies was similar, as shown in Table 4.2.

In the MRC study, pre-operative radiotherapy was allowed at the discretion of the treating clinician, whereas in the Intergroup study pre-operative radiotherapy was not permitted. Nine per cent of patients in each arm of the MRC study received pre-operative radiotherapy; however, exclusion of these patients did not change the observed effect of neoadjuvant chemotherapy on overall survival.

Other randomised controlled trials addressing this question have been published, but have enrolled only a few patients and so have been inadequately powered to detect a modest survival benefit favouring neoadjuvant chemotherapy. Two meta-analyses incorporating these trials have recently been published which also evaluated the role of neoadjuvant chemotherapy in localised oesophageal cancer. The Cochrane review (Malthaner et al. 2001) pooled the data from a total of seven randomised controlled trials, including 1,653 patients. The neoadjuvant chemotherapy arms all used cisplatin-based regimens, and patients who received radiotherapy in the two trials in which radiotherapy was allowed were excluded from the analysis. Significantly, two of the seven trials incorporated in this meta-analysis were the Intergroup 113 study and the MRC OEO2 study, which represented 1,267 patients. These two trials, also, were the only trials to include patients with adenocarcinoma of the oesophagus, in addition to squamous cell carcinoma. The pooled data showed no difference in mortality between the neoadjuvant chemotherapy and surgery alone arms at one year (odds ratio (OR) = 1.03), but at two years there was a 20% significant decrease in mortality favouring the neoadjuvant chemotherapy arm (OR = 0.80; 95% CI 0.65–0.99). There was a trend towards improved survival for neoadjuvant chemotherapy at three, four and five years.

The other meta-analysis (Urschel et al. 2002) pooled the data from a total of 11 randomised controlled trials, including 1,976 patients. As with the other meta-analysis, all patients who received pre-operative radiotherapy were excluded from the analysis. The pooled data showed no advantage for the neoadjuvant chemotherapy arm over the surgery alone arm, for 1-year survival (OR= 1.00; 95% CI 0.76–1.30; p = 0.98), 2-year survival (OR=0.88; 95% CI 0.62–1.24; p = 0.45), and 3-year survival (OR=0.77; 95% CI 0.37–1.59; p = 0.48). Those patients treated with surgery alone were more likely to have an oesophageal resection than those treated with neoadjuvant chemotherapy followed by surgery. Interestingly, however, the rate of complete (R0) resection was higher in those patients treated with neoadjuvant chemotherapy followed by surgery (OR=0.71; 95% CI 0.58–0.87; p = 0.001). Thirty-one per cent of patients had a clinical response to neoadjuvant chemotherapy, whereas a pathological complete response (pCR) was observed in 5%. There was no effect of neoadjuvant chemotherapy on the rate or pattern of cancer recurrence, either locoregional or distant. Importantly, this meta-analysis included two trials that did not report survival data, and survival data, in some instances, were obtained from graphically presented survival curves which are potentially subject to interpretation errors.

Based on the results of the MRC OEO2 study, the largest randomised controlled trial performed to address this issue so far, which showed a survival advantage for neoadjuvant chemotherapy followed by surgery, this has now been adopted as standard treatment in the UK and other parts of Europe. However, in North America, neoadjuvant chemotherapy is not routinely used, based on the negative results of the Intergroup 113 study.

Neoadjuvant chemotherapy in gastric cancer

So far, there have been no large, randomised controlled phase III trials comparing neoadjuvant chemotherapy followed by surgery versus surgery alone. However, numerous small phase II trials have been published, although direct comparisons between them cannot be made, as different inclusion criteria, staging methods and chemotherapy regimens were used. Table 4.3 summarises the results of eleven randomised trials that reported on survival. All trials contain a small number of patients, the largest including only 59 patients (Crookes *et al.* 1997), and so were not adequately powered to detect a survival benefit. Cisplatin-based chemotherapy regimens were used in all but two trials. Adjuvant chemotherapy was administered in seven trials, including intraperitoneal therapy in three trials. No radiotherapy was included in neoadjuvant or adjuvant treatment.

A recently published study (Lowy *et al.* 1999) pooled data from the three separate phase II trials conducted at the MD Anderson Cancer Centre, Houston, Texas, USA to evaluate whether a survival benefit existed with neoadjuvant chemotherapy. Eighty-three patients were evaluable who received one of three cisplatin-based neoadjuvant chemotherapy regimens (EFP, EAP, FIP). All resected patients underwent a total gastrectomy and D2 lymphadenectomy. Multivariate analysis of prognostic factors including T stage, nodal positivity, number of positive nodes and response to chemotherapy was performed, and only the response to chemotherapy was found to be significant (relative risk (RR) = 0.44; 95% CI 0.2–0.9; $p < 0.05$). Non-responders were found to have a median survival of 20 months, with a 5-year survival of 31%. In comparison, median survival for responders had not been reached at 26 months, and 5-year survival was 83%. The three patients who achieved a pCR were alive and disease-free at 48, 58 and 63 months post-surgery. Although these results are encouraging, they must be interpreted with caution, as the pooled results are from three non-randomised single institution studies. However, the sudies by Kelsen *et al.*

Table 4.3 Trials of neoadjuvant chemotherapy in gastric cancer

Reference	Neoadjuvant chemotherapy regimen	Adjuvant chemotherapy regimen	Radiotherapy	Number of patients	R0 resection rate	Number of pCRs	Median survival (months)	2 year survival rates	Comments
Wilke et al. 1989	EAP for 2 cycles	EAP for 2 cycles	No	34	29%	5	18	26%	Grade 3–4 neutropenia in 48% 1 toxic death
Ajani et al. 1991	EFP for 2 cycles	EFP for 3 cycles	No	25	72%	0	15	44%	1 postoperative death
Leichman et al. 1992	CF for 2 cycles	Intraperitoneal cisplatin/ floxuridine + IV sodium thiosulfate for 2 cycles	No	38	76%	3	17+	Not stated	Adjuvant IP therapy in 68% 1 toxic death
Ajani et al. 1993	EAP for 3 cycles	EAP for 2 cycles	No	48	77%	0	16	42%	Dose reduction in 77% 40% hospitalised with febrile neutropenia 1 toxic death
Rougier et al. 1994	CF for 1–6 cycles	Nil	No	30	59%	0	16	42%	1 toxic death Grade 4 neutropenia in 5 patients
Alexander et al. 1995	5FU/LV +IFN for 3 cycles	Nil	No	22	82%	0	18	52%	

contd.

EAP, etoposide, doxorubicin (Adriamycin), and cisplatin; EFP, etoposide, 5-fluorouracil, and cisplatin; CF, cisplatin, and 5-fluorouracil; 5FU/LV+IFN, 5-fluorouracil, leucovorin, and interferon; FAMTX, 5-fluorouracil, doxorubicin, and methotrexate; FUDR, 5-fluorodeoxyuridine; PLF, cisplatin, leucovorin, 5-fluorouracil.

Table 4.3 contd.

Reference	Neoadjuvant chemotherapy regimen	Adjuvant chemotherapy regimen	Radiotherapy	Number of patients	R0 resection rate	Number of pCRs	Median survival (months)	2 year survival rates	Comments
Kelsen et al. 1996	FAMTX for 3 cycles	Intraperitoneal CF + IV 5FU for 3 cycles	No	56	61%	Not stated 31 (for R0)	15	40%	60% had febrile neutropenia
Kang et al. 1996	EFP for 2-3 cycles vs surgery alone	EFP for 3-6 cycles vs surgery alone	No	53 / 54	71% / 61%	4 / 0	33 / 32	55% / 55%	In abstract form only No significant differences between the 2 arms
Crookes et al. 1997	CF for 2 cycles	Intraperitoneal FUDR/cisplatin for 1 cycle	No	59	71%	5	>48	64%	1 toxic death, 2 postoperative deaths ? earlier stage tumours over-represented
Ajani et al. 1999	CF+IFN for 5 cycles	Nil	No	30	83%	2	30 40 (for R0)	63%	47% received all 5 cycles
Fink ei al. 1999	PLF for 2 cycles	Nil	No	49	76%	0	36	62%	In abstract form only

EAP, etoposide, doxorubicin (Adriamycin), and cisplatin; EFP, etoposide, 5-fluorouracil, and cisplatin; CF, cisplatin, and 5-fluorouracil; 5FU/LV+IFN, 5-fluorouracil, leucovorin, and interferon; FAMTX, 5-fluorouracil, doxorubicin, and methotrexate; FUDR, 5-fluorodeoxyuridine; PLF, cisplatin, leucovorin, 5-fluorouracil.

(1996) and Ajani *et al.* (1999) reported median survival figures of 31–40 months for those patients who underwent R0 resections. In addition, the median survival for the same group of patients in the study by Fink *et al.* (1999) had not been reached after a median follow-up of 28 months.

These small studies suggest that survival appears to be enhanced by combination chemotherapy for those patients who achieve a pCR, and have a R0 resection performed. Effective combination chemotherapy regimens exist, with acceptable toxicity profiles that result in a significant (>10%) rate of pCR. Importantly, surgical morbidity and mortality is not compromised, and the delay in surgery does not adversely impact on the rate of R0 resections performed. However, there is currently insufficient evidence to recommend neoadjuvant chemotherapy outside of the clinical trial setting, and the need for large multicentre, prospective randomised trials is obvious.

The large United Kingdom Medical Research Council Adjuvant Gastric Infusional Chemotherapy ('MAGIC') trial, which evaluated the efficacy of peri-operative chemotherapy, has recently been reported (Allum *et al.* 2003). Five hundred and three patients with resectable adenocarcinoma of the stomach (74%), oesophagogastric junction (12%) and lower third of the oesophagus (14%) were randomly assigned to pre-operative chemotherapy followed by surgery, then post-operative chemotherapy or surgery alone. ECF consisting of epirubicin (50 mg/m^2), cisplatin (60 mg/m^2) and protracted venous infusion 5-FU (300 mg/m^2) was used in the peri-operative chemotherapy arm based on its activity in two large RCTs in advanced disease (Ross *et al.* 2002; Webb *et al.* 1997). Patient characteristics including age, sex, site, performance status and maximum tumour diameter prior to treatment were well balanced in both arms. Of those patients who underwent surgery resection was deemed curative in a higher proportion in the chemotherapy arm (79% compared to 69%, $p = 0.018$). Post-operative deaths and complications were similar in both arms. Downstaging of the tumour was demonstrated in the chemotherapy arm versus the surgery arm, with a significantly lower maximum resected tumour diameter (3.1cm compared to 5cm, $p<0.001$). With a median follow up of 2 years the progression free survival was significantly higher for the chemotherapy arm (HR 0.70 [95% CI: 0.56–0.88]. There was a trend towards superior median overall survival for the chemotherapy arm (HR 0.80, 95% CI: 0.63–1.01). Preliminary results showed that peri-operative chemotherapy was associated with significantly higher curative resection rates, significantly improved progression-free survival and a strong trend towards better survival compared with surgery alone. The early results from the MAGIC trial are compelling, especially taken in conjunction with the results of the MRC OEO2 study. Therefore, while awaiting the definitive results from the MAGIC study, some clinicians may elect to offer patients peri-operative chemotherapy.

The large randomised trial in advanced oesophagogastric cancer reported by Webb *et al.* (1997) and Waters *et al.* (1999) compared ECF with the standard combination of FAMTX in 274 patients. ECF was administered 3 weekly to a maximum of eight cycles, whereas FAMTX was given every 4 weeks to a maximum of six cycles. ECF resulted in a significantly better overall response rate (46% versus 21%; $p = 0.00003$), median survival (8.7 months versus 6.1 months; $p = 0.0005$), and 2-year survival (14% versus 5%; $p = 0.03$) compared with FAMTX. The toxicity profile also favoured ECF with less haematologic toxicity and infection, but more alopecia and emesis. Although ECF required a central venous catheter, complications requiring removal occurred in only 15% of patients, with none being life threatening or causing long-term morbidity. In addition, among the 19 patients who received neoadjuvant ECF and proceeded to surgery, 10 (53%) underwent a R0 resection and 3 had a pCR. In comparison, there was no pCR achieved with FAMTX.

The study reported by Ross *et al.* (2002) is the largest randomised trial in advanced oesophago-gastric cancer. Mitomycin C, which has shown significant activity in advanced colorectal cancer in combination with protracted venous infusion 5-fluorouracil (Ross *et al.* 1997), was substituted for epirubicin. A total of 580 patients were recruited and randomised to ECF given 3-weekly for a maximum of eight cycles or MCF given every 6 weeks for a maximum of four cycles. The overall response rate (ECF 42.4%; MCF 44.1%), median survival (7 months for both arms) and 1-year survival (ECF 40%; MCF 32.7%) were similar between the two arms. There was also little difference in toxicity; however, global quality-of-life scores favoured ECF at 3 and 6 months.

Therefore, on the basis of these two trials, ECF is now regarded as one of the standard regimens for advanced disease, and is now being actively studied in the neoadjuvant setting. The results for ECF in these two trials is summarised in Table 4.4.

Table 4.4 Results of ECF in randomised trials

	ECF vs FAMTX	ECF vs MCF
Number of patients in ECF arm	126	290
Response rate	45%	42%
95% confidence interval	0.36–0.54	0.37–0.48
Median survival	8.9 months	9.4 months
2-year survival	11%	16%

Future directions

In the UK, a new large randomised study of neoadjuvant chemotherapy in patients with resectable adenocarcinoma of the oesophagus is now underway. A planned recruitment of 1,300 patients will be randomised to either two cycles of cisplatin and 5-fluorouracil given according to the schedule used in the MRC OEO2 study, or four cycles of epirubicin, cisplatin and capecitabine, an oral fluoropyrimidine (ECX regimen) followed by surgery.

A randomised multicentre study (REAL 2) with a 2×2 factorial design to compare the efficacy of capecitabine with 5-fluorouracil, and oxaliplatin with cisplatin in the

ECF regimen, for patients with advanced oesophago-gastric cancer, is underway. Patients are randomised to one of four treatment arms including the standard epirubicin, cisplatin, 5-fluorouracil regimen (ECF), a regimen where oxaliplatin has been substituted for cisplatin (EOF), a regimen where 5-fluorouracil has been substituted by capecitabine (ECX), and a regimen where both oxaliplatin and capecitabine are used in combination with epirubicin (EOX). The study aims to enrol 600 patients and the primary endpoint will be 1-year survival. Preliminary results reported by Tebbutt *et al.* (2002) are summarised in Table 4.5, and showed anti-tumour activity for both capecitabine and oxaliplatin. This confirms the rationale for testing capecitabine in the neoadjuvant setting.

Table 4.5 REAL-2 study treatment responses

	5FU vs capecitabine		*Cisplatin vs oxaliplatin*	
	ECF/EOF	ECX/EOX	ECF/ECX	EOF/EOX
Number of patients	103	95	95	103
Complete response (%)	4 (3.9%)	5 (5.3%)	5 (5.3%)	4 (3.9%)
Partial response (%)	32 (31.1%)	34 (35.8%)	26 (27.4%)	40 (38.9%)
Stable disease (%)	44 (42.7%)	38 (40%)	41 (43.2%)	41 (39.8%)
Progressive disease (%)	23 (22.3%)	18 (18.9%)	23 (24.2%)	18 (17.5%)
Objective response rate (%)	35%	41.1%	32.6%	42.7%

For oxaliplatin, a recent small, non-randomised trial by Catalano *et al.* (2002) showed a 22% response rate in patients with advanced gastric cancer who had been previously treated with cisplatin-based chemotherapy. This potential lack of cross-resistance to oxaliplatin warrants further investigation in pre-treated and chemo-naïve patients. Table 4.6 summarises selected trials that evaluated oxaliplatin in advanced oesophago-gastric cancer.

Irinotecan, a semisynthetic topoisomerase I inhibitor, has been studied in several small trials in advanced oesophago-gastric cancer. As a single agent it has modest activity in chemo-naïve patients, with overall response rates of 15–20%, as reported by Kohne *et al.* (1999), Enzinger *et al.* (2000) and Lin *et al.* (2000). In combination therapy, irinotecan has been shown, in chemo-naïve patients, to have response rates of 18–62%, as summarised in Table 4.7. A randomised phase II study reported by Pozzo *et al.* (2000) showed improved survival for irinotecan in combination with 5-fluorouracil compared with the combination of irinotecan with cisplatin. In addition, Assersohn *et al.* (2002) reported that as second-line therapy after cisplatin and 5-fluorouracil, the combination of irinotecan and 5-fluorouracil showed a response rate of 20%. As a result of these encouraging response rates, the role of irinotecan in neoadjuvant chemotherapy, or chemo-radiotherapy, for oesophago-gastric cancer is undergoing further investigation in clinical trials.

Table 4.6 Selected published trials evaluating oxaliplatin in advanced oesophago-gastric cancer

Reference	Tumour site	Pre-treated	Number of patients	Treatment regimen	Response rate	Comments
Khushalani et al. 2002	Oesophagus	No	36	Oxaliplatin 85 mg/m^2 D1+15+29, 5-FU 180 mg/m^2/day D8-42, + concurrent radiotherapy + surgery (n = 13)	81% 38% pCR	Oxaliplatin dose escalation to 100 mg/m^2 not feasible
Tebbutt et al. 2002	Oesophagus, OGJ, and stomach	No	43	Epirubicin 50 mg/m^2, oxaliplatin 130 mg/m^2, 5-FU 200 mg/m^2/day or capecitabine 1000–1250 mg/m^2/day; cycle repeated every 3 weeks	48%	Results from interim analysis in abstract form only

Table 4.7 Selected published trials evaluating irinotecan in advanced oesophago-gastric cancer

Reference	Tumour site	Pre-treated	Number of patients	Treatment regimen	Response rate	Comments
Ilson *et al.* 1999	Oesophagus	No	35	Irinotecan 65 mg/m^2, cisplatin 30 mg/m^2 weekly × 4 every 6 weeks	57%	17% of patients hospitalised, most commonly for febrile neutropenia
Ilson *et al.* 1999	Stomach	No	14	Irinotecan 65 mg/m^2, cisplatin 30 mg/m^2 weekly × 4 every 6 weeks	18%	
Blanke *et al.* 2001	OGJ and stomach	No	36	Irinotecan 125 mg/m^2, 5-FU 500 mg/m^2, leucovorin 20 mg/m^2 weekly × 4 every 6 weeks	22%	3 toxic deaths from neutropenic sepsis
Ajani *et al.* 2002	OGJ and stomach	No	36	Irinotecan 65 mg/m^2, cisplatin 30 mg/m^2 weekly × 4 every 6 weeks	58%	1 toxic death Modification of dose/schedule suggested

OGJ, oesophagogastric junction.

Taxanes, such as paclitaxel and docetaxel, have been studied extensively both in pre-treated and chemo-naïve patients with oesophago-gastric cancer. Modest response rates ranging from 10–30% have been reported as a single agent, and numerous combination trials in advanced disease have been reported. These trials are summarised in Table 4.8. In the neoadjuvant setting, paclitaxel has been used in combination with cisplatin (with or without 5-fluorouracil) and radiotherapy, with impressive pCR rates of 23–30% having been reported by Ajani *et al.* (2001) and Bains *et al.* (2002). These results are summarised in Table 4.9. As a result, the role of paclitaxel in neoadjuvant chemotherapy, both combined and in sequential fashion, is being further evaluated in clinical trials.

For docetaxel, similar reponse rates to paclitaxel of 5–20% have been reported as a single agent. Preliminary data from a study comparing docetaxel/cisplatin/5–FU (DCF) and 5–FU/cisplatin (FUP) have shown a survival benefit for DCF although there are some concerns with the preliminary haematological toxicity data (Ajani *et al.* 2003). In this preliminary analysis including only less than half of the patients recruited in the study, 111 patients were randomly assigned to DCF and 112 patients to FUP. The median survival was 10.2 months in the DCF arm and 8.5 months in the FUP arm ($p = 0.0064$).

Novel agents including matrix metalloproteinase (MMP) inhibitors and epithelial-derived growth factor receptor (EGFR) targeted therapies are being investigated in oesophago-gastric cancer. MMPs are a family of enzymes capable of degrading extra-cellular matrix, thus facilitating the invasion of malignant cells through connective tissue and blood vessel walls. Over-expression is associated with tumour metastatic potential. A study by Fielding *et al.* (2000) involved 369 patients with inoperable gastric cancer, and randomised them to marimastat, a MMP inhibitor, or placebo. A trend towards better median survival favoured marimstat (167 days versus 135 days; $p = 0.07$), and subgroup analysis revealed significantly improved survival in patients with advanced disease only without distant metastases (246 days versus 183 days; $p = 0.022$), and with prior chemotherapy (254 days versus 180 days; $p = 0.045$).

EGFR signalling pathways influence cell differentiation, proliferation, migration, angiogenesis, and apoptosis. An EGFR humanised, monoclonal antibody, cetuximab, has been shown in phase I trials to be well tolerated, with promising activity in various solid tumours. Phase I trials of cetuximab in combination with chemo-radiotherapy are underway in oesophageal cancer. In addition, a trial combining cetuximab with ECF chemotherapy is also ongoing. Oral EGFR tyrosine kinase inhibitors, namely ZD 1839 and OSI 774, are also being evaluated in oesophago-gastric cancer, and results of these trials are eagerly awaited.

Conclusions

There is clearly an emerging role for perioperative chemotherapy in oesophago-gastric cancer with, in the case of oesophageal cancer, the survival benefit of neoadjuvant chemotherapy being demonstrated in the largest randomised trial

Table 4.8 Selected published trials evaluating paclitaxel in advanced oesophago-gastric cancer

Reference	Tumour site	Pre-treated	Number of patients	Treatment regimen	Response rate	Comments
Ajani et al. 1994	Oesophagus	No	50	Paclitaxel 250 mg/m² + G-CSF; cycle repeated every 3 weeks	32%	
Ilson et al. 1998	Oesophagus	No	61	Paclitaxel 175 mg/m² D1, cisplatin15–20 mg/m²/day D1–5, 5-FU 750–1000 mg/m²/day D1–5, cycle repeated every 4 weeks	48%	48% hospitalised for mortality 11% toxic deaths 5-FU dose attenuated after severe toxicity in the first 10 patients
Ilson et al. 2000	Oesophagus, and OGJ	No	38	Paclitaxel 200–250 mg/m² over 24 hours D1, cisplatin 75 mg/m² D2 + G-CSF, cycle repeated every 3 weeks	44%	50% hospitalised for toxicity 11% toxic deaths
Polee et al. 2002	Oesophagus, and OGJ	No	51	Paclitaxel 180 mg/m² D1, cisplatin 60 mg/m² D1, cycle repeated every 2 weeks	43%	

G-CSF, granulocyte colony-stimulating factor.

Table 4.9 Selected published trials evaluating neoadjuvant treatment with paclitaxel in localised oesophago-gastric cancer

Reference	Tumour site	Number of patients	Treatment regimen	Response rate	Comments
Ajani et al. 2001	Oesophagus, and OGJ	37	Paclitaxel 200 mg/m^2 over 24 hours D1, cisplatin 15 mg/m^2/day D1–5, 5-FU 750 mg/m^2/day D1–5, cycle repeated every 4 weeks for 2 cycles followed by concurrent CRT followed by surgery (n = 35)	30%	pCR 2 postoperative deaths
Bains et al. 2002	Oesophagus	41	Paclitaxel 175 mg/m^2 D1, cisplatin 75 mg/m^2 D1, followed by concurrent CRT followed by surgery (n = 33)	26%	pCR 2 postoperative deaths

CRT, chemoradiotherapy

Table 4.10 Selected published trials evaluating docetaxel in advanced oesophago-gastric cancer

Reference	Tumour site	Pre-treated	Number of patients	Treatment regimen	Response rate	Comments
Einzig et al. (1996)	OGJ, and stomach	No	41	Docetaxel 100 mg/m^2 D1 every 3 weeks	17%	
Heath et al. (2002)	Oesophagus	Yes/no	22	Docetaxel 75 mg/m^2 D1 every 3 weeks	18%	Responses seen in chemo-naïve patients only

reported so far. The integration of new targeted therapies shows promise and could further improve outcome. There is a divergence of treatment paradigm between North America and the UK for localised oesophageal cancer. Neoadjuvant chemotherapy is standard treatment in the UK, whereas in North America patients receive surgery alone or definitive chemo-radiotherapy. The role of neoadjuvant chemotherapy in gastric cancer remains to be defined, and the final results of the MAGIC study are eagerly awaited. Furthermore, the forthcoming MRC OEO 5 study should provide additional information. New drugs including capecitabine, oxaliplatin, irinotecan, and taxanes are being tested in the neoadjuvant setting having shown significant activity in advanced disease. Optimal integration of these drugs and targeted therapies into peri-operative treatment may improve the poor prognosis of oesophago-gastric cancer in the future.

References

Ajani, J. A., Ota, D. M., Jessop, J. M. *et al.* (1991). Resectable gastric carcinoma. An evaluation of preoperative and postoperative chemotherapy. *Cancer* **68**, 1501–1506.

Ajani, J. A., Mayer, R. J., Ota, D. M., *et al.* (1993). Preoperative and postoperative combination chemotherapy for potentially resectable gastric carcinoma. *Journal of the National Cancer Institute* **85**, 1839–1844.

Ajani, J. A., Ilson, D. H., Daugherty, K. *et al.* (1994). Activity of taxol in patients with squamous cell carcinoma and adenocarcinoma of the esophagus. *Journal of the National Cancer Institute* **86**, 1086–1091.

Ajani, J. A., Mansfield, P. F., Lynch, P. M. *et al.* (1999). Enhanced staging and all chemotherapy preoperatively in patients with potentially resectable gastric carcinoma. *Journal of Clinical Oncology* **17**, 2403–2411.

Ajani, J. A., Komaki, R., Putnam, J. B. *et al.* (2001). A three-step strategy of induction chemotherapy then chemoradiation followed by surgery in patients with potentially resectable carcinoma of the esophagus or gastroesophageal junction. *Cancer* **92**, 279–286.

Ajani, J. A., Baker, J, Pisters, P. W. *et al.* (2002). CPT-11 plus cisplatin in patients with advanced, untreated gastric or gastroesophageal junction carcinoma: results of a phase II study. *Cancer* **94**, 641–646.

Ajani, J. A., Van Cutsem, E., Moiseyenko, V., Tjulandin, S., Fodor, M., Majlis, M., Boni, C., Zuber, E. & Blattmann, A. (2003). Docetaxel, cisplatin, 5–fluorouracil compare to cisplatin and 5–fluorouracil for chemotherapy-naive patients with metastatic or locally recurrent unresectable gastric carcinoma: interim results of a randomized phase III trial (V325). *Proceedings of the American Society of Clinical Oncology* **22**, 249.

Alexander, H. R., Grem, J. L., Hamilton, J. M. *et al.* (1995). Thymidylate synthase protein expression. *Cancer Journal of Scientific America* **1**, 49.

Allgayer, H., Babic, R., Gruetzner, K. U. *et al.* (2000). c-erbB-2 is of independent prognostic relevance in gastric cancer and is associated with the expression of tumor-associated protease systems. *Journal of Clinical Oncology* **18**, 2201–2209.

Allum, W. H., Cunningham, D. & Weeden, S. (2003). Perioperative chemotherapy in operable gastric and lower oesophageal cancer: a randomised, controlled trial (the MAGIC trial, ISRCRN 93793971). *Proceedings of the American Society of Clinical Oncology* **22**, 249.

Assersohn, L., Rigg, A., Cunningham, D. *et al.* (2002). A phase II trial of irinotecan and 5-fluorouracil (5FU) and folinic acid (FA) in patients with oesophago-gastric carcinoma who had progressed or relapsed within 3 months of 5FU-based chemotherapy. *Proceedings of the American Society of Clinical Oncology* **21**, 157a (abstract 625).

Bains, M. S., Stojadinovic, A., Minsky, B. *et al.* (2002). A phase II trial of preoperative combined-modality therapy for localized esophageal carcinoma: initial results. *Journal of Cardiovascular Surgery* **124**, 270–277.

Blanke, C. D., Haller, D. G., Benson, A. B. *et al.* (2001). A phase II study of irinotecan with 5-fluorouracil and leucovorin in patients with previously untreated gastric adenocarcinoma. *Annals of Oncology* **12**, 1575–1580.

Catalano, V., Graziano, F., Salvagni, S. *et al.* (2002). Lack of resistance to oxaliplatin (l-OHP) based chemotherapy in patients with advanced gastric cancer previously treated with cisplatin-containing regimens: preliminary results of a phase II study. *Proceedings of the American Society of Clinical Oncology* **21**, 97b (abstract 2200).

Crookes, P., Leichman, C. G., Leichman, L. *et al.* (1997). Systemic chemotherapy for gastric carcinoma followed by postoperative intraperitoneal therapy: a final report. *Cancer* **79**, 1767–1775.

Enzinger, P. C., Kulke, M. H., Clark, J. W. *et al.* (2000). A phase II trial of CPT-11 in previouly untreated patients with advanced adenocarcinoma of the esophagus and stomach. *Proceedings of the American Society of Clinical Oncology* **19**, 315a (abstract 1243).

Einzig, A. I., Neuberg, D., Remick, S. C. *et al.* (1996). Phase II trial of docetaxel (Taxotere) in patients with adenocarcinoma of the upper gastrointestinal tract previously untreated with cytotoxic chemotherapy: the Eastern Cooperative Oncology Group (ECOG) results of protocol E1293. *Medical Oncology* **13**, 87–93.

Ferlay, J., Bray, F., Pisani, P. *et al.* (2001). *GLOBOCAN 2000 – Cancer Incidence, Mortality, and Prevalence Worldwide. Version 1.0.*

Fielding, J., Schofield, J., Stuart R. *et al.* (2000). A randomized double-blind placebo-controlled study of Marimastat in patients with inoperable gastric adenocarcinoma. *Proceedings of the American Society of Clinical Oncology* **19**, 240a (abstract 929).

Fink, U., Ott, K., Dittler, H. J. *et al.* (1999). Neoadjuvant cisplatinum, leucovorin and fluorouracil (PLF) in adequately staged patients with locally advanced gastric carcinoma. *Proceedings of the American Society of Clinical Oncology* **18**, 272a (abstract 1044).

Heath, E. I., Urba, S., Marshall, J. *et al.* (2002). A phase II trial of docetaxel chemotherapy in patients with incurable adenocarcinoma of the esophagus. *Investigation of New Drugs* **20**, 95–99.

Ilson, D. H., Ajani, J. A., Bhalla, K. *et al.* (1998). Phase II trial of paclitaxel, fluorouracil, and cisplatin in patients with advanced carcinoma of the esophagus. *Journal of Clinical Oncology* **16**, 1826–1834.

Ilson, D. H., Saltz, L., Enzinger, P. *et al.* (1999). Phase II trial of weekly irinotecan plus cisplatin in advanced esophageal cancer. *Journal of Clinical Oncology* **17**, 3270–3275.

Ilson, D. H., Enzinger, P., Saltz, L. *et al.* (1999). Phase II trial of weekly irinotecan + cisplatin in advanced gastric cancer. *Proceedings of the American Society of Clinical Oncology* **18**, 259a (abstract 994).

Ilson, D. H., Forastiere, A., Arquette, M. *et al.* (2000). A phase II trial of paclitaxel and cisplatin in patients with advanced carcinoma of the esophagus. *Journal of Cancer* **6**, 316–323.

Kang, Y. K., Choi, D. W., Im, Y. H. *et al.* (1996). A phase III randomized comparison of neoadjuvant chemotherapy followed by surgery versus surgery for locally advanced stomach cancer. *Proceedings of the American Society of Clinical Oncology* **15**, 215 (abstract 503).

Katano, M., Nakamura, M., Fujimoto, K. *et al.* (1998). Prognostic value of platelet-derived growth factor-A (PDGF-A) in gastric carcinoma. *Annals of Surgery* **227**, 365–371.

Kelsen, D. P., Karpeh, M., Schwartz, G. *et al.* (1996). Neoadjuvant therapy for high risk gastric cancer: a phase II trial of preoperative FAMTX and postoperative intraperitoneal fluorouracil-cisplatin plus intravenous fluorouracil. *Journal of Clinical Oncology* **14**, 1818–1828.

Kelsen, D. P., Ginsberg, R., Pajak, T. F. *et al.* (1998). Chemotherapy followed by surgery compared with surgery alone for localized esophageal cancer. *New England Journal of Medicine* **339**, 1979–1984.

Kelsen, D. P., Pajak, T. F. & Ginsberg, R. (1999). Treatment of esophageal cancer. *New England Journal of Medicine* **340**, 1685–1687.

Khushalani, N. I., Leichman, C. G., Proulx, G. *et al.* (2002). Oxaliplatin in combination with protracted-infusion fluorouracil and radiation: report of a clinical trial for patients with esophageal cancer. *Journal of Clinical Oncology* **20**, 2844–2850.

Kohne, C. H., Thuss-Patience, P., Catane, R. *et al.* (1999). Final results of a phase II trial of CPT-11 in patients with advanced gastric cancer. *Proceedings of the American Society of Clinical Oncology* **18**, 258a (abstract 993).

Kuwahara, A., Katano, M., Nakamura, M. *et al.* (1999). New therapeutic strategy for gastric carcinoma: a two-step evaluation of malignant potential from its molecular biologic and pathologic characteristics. *Journal of Surgical Oncology* **72**, 142–149.

Leichman, L., Silberman, H., Leichman, C. G. *et al.* (1992). Preoperative systemic chemotherapy followed by adjuvant postoperative intraperitoneal therapy for gastric cancer: a University of Southern California pilot program. *Journal of Clinical Oncology* **10**, 1933–1942.

Lin, L. & Hecht, J. R. (2000). A phase II trial of irinotecan in patients with advanced adenocarcinoma of the gastroesophageal (GE) junction. *Proceedings of the American Society of Clinical Oncology* **19**, 289a (abstract 1130).

Lowy, A. M., Mansfield, P. F., Leach, S. D. *et al.* (1999). Response to neoadjuvant chemotherapy best predicts survival after curative resection of gastric cancer. *Annals of Surgery* **229**, 303–308.

Malthaner, R. & Fenlon, D. (2001). Preoperative chemotherapy for resectable thoracic esophageal cancer (Cochrane Review). *The Cochrane Library* **1**, CD001556.

Medical Research Council Oesophageal Cancer Working Party (2002). Surgical resection with or without preoperative chemotherapy in oesophageal cancer: A randomised controlled trial. *The Lancet* **359**, 1727–1733.

Metzger, R., Leichman, C. G., Danenberg, K. D. *et al.* (1998). ERCC-1 mRNA levels complement thymidylate synthase mRNA levels in predicting response and survival for gastric cancer patients receiving combination cisplatin and fluorouracil chemotherapy. *Journal of Clinical Oncology* **16**, 309–316.

Miyata, H., Doki, Y., Shiozaki, H. *et al.* (2000). CDC25B and p53 are independently implicated in radiation sensitivity for human esophageal cancers. *Clinical Cancer Research* **6**, 4859–4865.

Polee, M. B., Verweij, J., Siersema, P. D. *et al.* (2002). Phase I study of a weekly schedule of a fixed dose of cisplatin and escalating doses of paclitaxel in patients with advanced oesophageal cancer. *European Journal of Cancer* **38**, 1495–1500.

Pozzo, J., Szanto, C., Peschel, T. *et al.* (2000). Multicentric randomized phase II trial of irinotecan (IRI) in combination with cisplatin (C) or with 5-fluorouracil (FU) and folinic acid (FA) in patients with advanced gastric or GE-junction adenocarcinoma (AGC-AGEJC). *Proceedings of the American Society of Clinical Oncology* **19**, 303a (abstract 1190).

Ross, P., Norman, A., Cunningham, D. *et al.* (1997). A prospective randomized trial of protracted venous infusion (PVI) 5-FU with or without mitomycin C (MMC) in advanced colorectal cancer. *Annals of Oncology* **8**, 95–101.

Ross, P., Nicolson, M., Cunningham, D., Valle, J., Seymour, M., Harper, P., Price, T., Anderson, H., Iveson, T., Hickish, T., Lofts, F. & Norman, A. (2002). Prospective randomized trial comparing mitomycin, cisplatin, and protracted venous-infusion fluorouracil (PVI 5-FU) with epirubicin, cisplatin, and PVI 5-FU in advanced esophagogastric cancer. *Journal of Clinical Oncology* **20**, 1996–2004.

Rougier, P., Mahjoubi, M., Lasser, P. *et al.* (1994). Neoadjuvant chemotherapy in locally advanced gastric carcinoma – a phase II trial with combined continuous intravenous 5-fluorouracil and bolus cisplatinum. *European Journal of Cancer* **30A**, 1269–1275.

Schneider, P. M., Stoeltzing, O., Roth, J. A. *et al.* (2000). p53 mutational status improves estimation of prognosis in patients with curatively resected adenocarcinoma in Barrett's esophagus. *Clinical Cancer Research* **6**, 3153–3158.

Shih, C. H., Ozawa, S., Ando, N. *et al.* (2000). Vascular endothelial growth factor expression predicts outcome and lymph node metastasis in squamous cell carcinoma of the esophagus. *Clinical Cancer Research* **6**, 1161–1168.

Tebbutt, N., Norman, A., Cunningham, D. *et al.* (2002). Randomised, multicentre phase III study comparing capecitabine with fluorouracil and oxaliplatin with cisplatin in patients with advanced oesophago-gastric cancer; interim analysis. *Proceedings of the American Society of Clinical Oncology* **21**, 131a (abstract 523).

Urschel, J. D., Vasan, H. & Blewett, C. J. (2002). A meta-analysis of randomized controlled trials that compared neoadjuvant chemotherapy and surgery to surgery alone for resectable esophageal cancer. *American Journal of Surgery* **183**, 274–279.

Vizcaino, A. P., Moreno, V., Lambert, R. *et al.* (2002). Time trends incidence of both major histologic types of esophageal carcinomas in selected countries, 1973–1995. *International Journal of Cancer* **99**, 860–868.

Waters, J. S., Norman, A., Cunningham, D. *et al.* (1999). Long-term survival after epirubicin, cisplatin and fluorouracil for gastric cancer: results of a randomized trial. *British Journal of Cancer* **80**, 269–272.

Webb, A., Cunningham, D., Scarffe, J. H., Harper, P., Norman, A., Joffe, J. K., Hughes, M., Mansi, J., Findlay, M., Hill, A., Oates, J., Nicolson, M., Hickish, T. M. O., Iveson, T., Watson, M., Underhill, C., Wardley, A. & Meehan, M. (1997). Randomized trial comparing epirubicin, cisplatin, and fluorouracil versus fluorouracil, doxorubicin, and methotrexate in advanced esophagogastric cancer. *Journal of Clinical Oncology* **15**, 261–267.

Wilke, H., Preusser, P., Fink, U. *et al.* (1989). Preoperative chemotherapy in locally advanced and nonresectable gastric cancer: a phase II study with etoposide, doxorubicin, and cisplatin. *Journal of Clinical Oncology* **7**, 1318–1326.

Chapter 5

The role of pre-operative and definitive chemoradiation in oesophageal cancer

Adrian Crellin

Introduction

The literature on the optimal management of oesophageal cancer, and in particular the role of multimodality therapy, is complex and sometimes contradictory. The overall outlook for many patients with this disease is poor, owing to advanced stage at presentation. It is therefore not surprising that the results of surgery as a single treatment modality are disappointing. Radiotherapy, and more recently chemoradiation (CRT), has been used in the treatment of oesophageal cancer for many years. Oesophageal cancer is relatively chemo-sensitive with good response rates, and there is an established role for palliative chemotherapy. Why then is the role of these two modalities in the potentially curative setting not clearer?

The answer lies in difficulties interpreting trials, criticisms of the methodology or quality assurance within some trials, and so a lack of acceptance of the results. Many trials have been small. The complexity of different treatment regimes and the key relationship with surgery, coupled with variable toxicity have also made comparison between trials difficult. Many early trials have poor staging by modern standards and it is by no means certain which patients were included or that the arms of small randomized studies were well balanced. 'Single modality thinking' has meant that results have often not been viewed as a whole package of care, with a trade-off in terms of toxicities and improved overall outcomes. Vital questions about which sub-groups of patients may benefit from more complex treatments are unanswered.

Future studies should benefit from improved staging so that patients with metastatic disease are not included in trials of potentially curative therapy, but render comparisons with historical series impossible. The routine use of spiral computed tomography (CT) and the increasing access to endoscopic ultrasound (EUS) are part of the improved quality assurance in staging. There is also literature to suggest that additional patients with occult stage IV disease may be identified with routine isotope bone scans (13%) (Lamb *et al.* 2002) and positron emission tomography (PET) (14%) (Flamen *et al.* 2000).

An analysis of patterns of treatment failure is essential to look beneath overall survival outcomes to try to select specific groups of patients for specific therapies. Local relapse is a significant component of failure after surgery, and data on improved surgical quality assurance, with pathology verification, may be important in looking at future strategies. The high distant metastatic failure rate means that systemic therapy will need to be a key component in improving outcomes.

Preoperative chemoradiation

There is an increasing concentration on pre-operative therapy in the treatment of both oesophageal and pancreatic cancer. The scale of the operation means that a significant proportion of patients may have a significant recovery period with complications, leading to a poor uptake or delay of post-operative therapy. The post-operative component of chemotherapy was not accessed in 32% of patients in the American Intergroup trial INT 0113 (Kelsen *et al.* 1998) and in 40% in an interim report of the Medical Research Council (MRC) MAGIC study. Any strategy that effectively excludes patient numbers of this order is unlikely to be successful.

The use of concurrent chemotherapy and radiotherapy is attractive because it delivers enhanced local therapy and can potentially deliver neoadjuvant systemic therapy.

Non-randomised studies have provided some evidence of a significant change in the pattern of outcome from surgical resection alone, including a proportion of pathological complete responses (pCRs) (Mandard *et al.* 1994). There has been a pattern of increased toxicity, of variable severity. Forastiere *et al.* (1993) reported a series of 47 patients, of mixed squamous and adenocarcinoma histology, using 5-fluorouracil (5-FU), cisplatin and vinblastine with 37.5–45 Gy of radiotherapy. A transhiatal oesophagectomy was performed. No residual tumour was found in 24% of the resection specimens. The median survival was 29 months and there was no significant difference between adenocarcinoma and squamous histology. There was a big difference in 5-year survival based on pCR (60%) or not (32%). In addition, there were no local recurrences, in marked contrast to 23% in a previous trial.

Much of the non-randomised literature since then has reproduced results with great promise, variable levels of toxicity and pCR rates up to 50%. However, it is important to look critically at these figures as different denominators are used based on: numbers of operations, successful resections, primary tumour specimens, or intent to treat. However, consistent figures of 20–30% are achieved, which is significantly higher than chemotherapy alone as a single modality. There are many phase II studies reported in the literature using different drug combinations and radiotherapy doses (Geh *et al.* 2001). However, this generation of studies and the randomised trials are dominated by cisplatin and 5FU combinations.

The most important randomised studies are seen in Table 5.1. Earlier trials used sequential chemotherapy with radiotherapy following, both given as separate modalities. Later trials used true concurrent chemotherapy and radiotherapy with the modalities given at the same time. There is evidence that this is potentially beneficial in terms of response rates, but toxicity can be increased. Some trials are small and are underpowered.

Table 5.1 Randomised trials of pre-operative chemoradiotherapy

Reference	Sequential or concurrent	Squamous and/or adeno.	Number of patients	Chemotherapy	Radiotherapy dose (Gy)	Resection rate	Post-operative mortality CRT	Result
Nygard et al. 1992	S	S	88	Cis/Bleo	35	66%	24%	Negative
Le Prise et al. 1994	S	S	86	Cis/5FU	20	85%	8%	Negative
Bosset et al. 1997	S	S	282	Cis	37	78%	12%	Improved Disease Free Survival
Apinop et al. 1994	C	S	69	Cis/5FU	40	74%	12%	Negative
Walsh et al. 1996	C	A	113	Cis/5FU	40	90%	10%	Improved overall survival
Urba et al. 2001	C	A/s	100	Cis/5FU/Vinbl	45	–	–	Negative
Burmeister et al. 2002	C	A/s	256	Cis/5FU	35	85%	6.4%	Negative

Bosset reported the results of a randomised trial of 282 patients (Bosset *et al.* 1997). It included only squamous carcinoma and had CT staging. Cisplatin at a dose of 80mg/m^2 was given for two courses followed very closely by a split course of radiotherapy of 18.5 Gy in five fractions repeated after two weeks. Surgery, a radical two stage resection, was performed four weeks after the last fraction. The control arm went straight to surgery. There was no difference in overall survival between the arms although there was a significant difference in the disease-free survival. A significant increase in post-operative mortality of 12.3% versus 3.6% reduced the survival benefit from the treatment. The complications were largely respiratory and infective. The high radiotherapy dose per fraction may have contributed to the morbidity. However, in follow up, the cancer cause of death rates were significantly different (86.1% versus 67.6%, $p = 0.002$), favouring the combined modality arm.

The most influential and also controversial study has been the 'Walsh' trial (Walsh *et al.* 1996). This led to pre-operative CRT being adopted as a standard of care in the USA. It was an interim analysis of 113 patients, reporting only those with adenocarcinoma. There was no CT staging. The control arm had surgery alone, with the novel arm receiving two courses of cisplatin and 5FU with one of these being given concurrently with 40 Gy in 15 fractions of radiotherapy. The radiotherapy technique was unsophisticated by modern standards and may have contributed to the significant morbidity. The results at 3 years showed a significant improvement in survival in favour of the combined treatment arm (32% versus 6%, $p = 0.01$). Criticisms of this trial have centred on the method of analysis and the extraordinarily poor survival in the control arm. Attempts to implement this regime in the UK more widely have encountered quite marked toxicity.

A University of Michigan trial of 100 patients using a cisplatin/5FU/vinblastine combination with 45 Gy in 30 fractions of radiotherapy initially showed no survival difference compared with transhiatal surgery alone (Urba *et al.* 2001). Results reported at 3 years in 1997 demonstrated a survival difference that disappeared when the final results appeared in 2001. This trial was only powered to detect a large difference in survival which was seen in a preliminary non-randomised study. The survival curves show clearly the improvement in outcome in those demonstrating a marked pathological response, which is common feature of many chemoradiotherapy trials.

The most recent, and very important, trial was reported by Burmeister at the American Society of Clinical Oncology meeting in 2002 (Burmeister *et al.* 2002). It was a collaborative Trans-Tasman Radiation Oncology Group (TROG) and Australasian Gastro-Intestinal Trials Group (AGITG) randomized study of 256 patients. The tumours were adenocarcinoma in 61%, and patients were well staged. They received one course of cisplatin/5FU and 35 Gy of radiotherapy followed by surgery, compared with surgery alone. There was no difference in overall survival. There have been criticisms that the doses of chemotherapy and radiotherapy were low.

The quality of surgery was high and the results of the surgery alone arm good. Importantly, data were presented demonstrating a big difference in the outcome with histology. Those patients with squamous tumours had a significant increase in path CR (26.3% squamous versus 9.0% adenocarcinoma), an improved overall survival and significantly improved disease-free survival compared with control.

There have been problems in the quality assurance or technical delivery of the three treatments, leading to difficulties in interpreting many studies. The issue of balancing toxicity and improvements in outcome has been difficult to quantify. A combined Leeds and Bristol phase II study CARE (chemotherapy and radiotherapy with excision) was designed to pilot and assess the tolerability of optimised pre-op chemotherapy, conformal radiotherapy and radical two-stage surgery in well-staged patients with a parallel quality-of-life study and good pathology. The results will be published shortly but show a good resection rate (76%) with a path CR rate of 21% and a post-operative mortality rate of 6.4%. There was significant toxicity, particularly in intensifying the chemotherapy, and in using infusion 5FU. A regime using cisplatin and paclitaxel with 50.4 Gy at the Memorial Sloane Kettering Caner Center, New York (Bains *et al.* 2002) can produce similar results but without line related complications and all treatment given as an outpatient.

With the results of the MRC OEO2 Trial showing a significant improvement in survival (43% versus 34%) at 2 years (MRC Oesophagus Working Group 2002) with a relatively well-tolerated short cisplatin/5FU regime, there would need to be a marked increase in benefit and further evidence to justify the use of chemoradiotherapy pre-operatively, given the increase in toxicity. More trials will be needed to optimise chemotherapy. The OEO2 results suggest that the mechanism of action may have been to downstage the tumours, allowing a higher rate of successful resection rather than to affect death with metastatic disease. Longer-term results will need to be awaited, but the patterns of recurrence will be important. Thus optimising surgery and predicting salvageable local failures as well as trying to influence systemic failure will be the scope for future studies. It may be that selected patients who have positive resection margins, who have a poorer outlook, should still have CRT, as in rectal cancer, if they could be predicted. Local recurrence may still be a significant cause of failure and there is evidence of the use of post-operative radiotherapy in oesophageal (Xiao *et al.* 2003) or CRT in gastric cancer to improve results (Macdonald *et al.* 2001).

The increase in incidence of adenocarcinoma arising at the gastro-oesophageal junction, and evidence of good results with chemoradiation alone in squamous cancer, have led to a separation of trials for these two diseases.

Definitive chemoradiation

Radical radiotherapy has been a treatment option for localised non-metastatic oesophageal carcinoma for many years. It has been particularly used in squamous cancer. The question of whether the addition of chemotherapy, given concurrently, improves the results has been important. There is no doubt that the toxicity is higher and that the current spectrum of drugs rules out some patients because of age or coincident benign conditions.

The most important trial has been the 'Herskovic' study (Al-Sarraf *et al.* 1997). A total of 123 patients were randomised to receive either radiotherapy alone to a dose of 64 Gy or two courses of cisplatin and infusional 5FU concurrent with 50 Gy of radiotherapy. Two more courses of chemotherapy were scheduled after the completion of the radiotherapy. The initial radiotherapy fields covered extended nodal target volumes to 30 Gy. There was a significant benefit in 2- and 5-year survival (36% and 30% CRT versus 10% and 0% RT, respectively). The rate of distant metastatic disease was reduced in the combined modality arm (12% versus 26%). The survival curve was flat after 2.5 years, implying that long-term survival is an achievable goal for some patients.

In a confirmatory study, 69 non-randomised patients were treated with the CRT protocol, achieving similar results in terms of median survival and with a 3-year survival of 26%. The acute toxicity in the combined treatment arm was significantly higher with notably myelosuppression renal impairment and mucositis as the major problems. There was no significant difference in the late complication rates. Relatively poor overall survival in the radiotherapy alone control arm remains a question mark against the study.

The Cochrane review of chemoradiotherapy versus radiotherapy in 13 trials has confirmed that there is a benefit to combined modality therapy with a reduction in mortality of 9% and an improved local control rate of 5% (Wong *et al.* 2002). It is at the expense of increased toxicity.

There is no doubt, however, that with careful selection and high-quality treatment delivery, good results can be achieved with radiotherapy alone (Sykes *et al.* 1998). Radical treatment should not be ruled out if the chemotherapy component represents too high a risk.

The results with both squamous and adenocarcinoma appear to be similar. Many UK centres have experience in treating patients who have localised disease, but because of coincident medical conditions ruling out surgery, age or patient choice. The results appear reproducible with this 'selected' group, with survival being in the region of 35% at 2 years, comparable to the surgery alone control arm in the MRC OEO2 study.

It is in the squamous tumours that chemoradiotherapy may prove a viable alternative to surgical resection. There is accumulating evidence of outcomes equivalent to surgery, stage by stage (Chan *et al.* 1999). The important trial of chemoradiotherapy versus surgery may be difficult to do because of patient numbers, even in a collaborative multi-national setting. The older age and position of the disease within the chest may also mean that the question may become whether there is a role for surgical salvage in selected patients after failure of CRT.

What can be done to improve the outcomes of chemoradiation?

The high local failure rate of 45% in the Herskovic trial led to the Intergroup study 0122 (Minsky *et al.* 1999), where the dose of external beam radiotherapy was increased to 64.8 Gy and the intensity of the chemotherapy increased in this 45 patient toxicity and survival phase II study. The results showed increased toxicity, with 11% treatment-related deaths compared with 2% in the Herskovic study. The protocol was not adopted into a phase III study. Another approach to improved local control was to use brachytherapy to intensify the radiotherapy dose to the tumour. Study RTOG 92-07 (Gaspar *et al.* 1997) used the 50 Gy external beam and chemotherapy protocol from the Herskovic protocol and added an intraluminal brachytherapy boost with one of two methods of delivery, high dose rate or low dose rate. Six of the 35 patients developed an oesophageal fistula. This toxicity was deemed unacceptable.

The technology and sophistication of radiotherapy delivery is changing at a fast pace. The use of spiral-CT-based imaging planning, enhanced with EUS information, allows more accurate delineation of the tumour and target volume. At the same time the ability to shape fields and treatment volumes allows potentially higher doses to the tumour with reduced normal tissue toxicity. The implementation of intensity modulated radiotherapy (IMRT) will allow better definition of radiotherapy dose and again improve the therapeutic ratio. Renewed interest in high light energy transfer (LET) particle therapies with protons and carbon ions may open completely different opportunities for non-surgical therapy, with promising results already seen in non-small-cell lung cancer (Miyamoto *et al.* 2003).

There is no doubt that many improvements will come from combining improved technical radiotherapy with systemic therapies. New combinations of radiation sensitising chemotherapeutic agents could improve response rates. Drugs such as cisplatin/paclitaxel, oxaliplatin/capecitabine, irinotecan and gemcitabine are all candidates for studies. Better toxicity profiles, greater convenience or minor improvements in response rates will be achieved in the next few years. The application of molecular biology and greater understanding of tumour biology holds promise. There is good evidence for direct cytotoxic and radiosensitising effects of tumour-necrosis factor (TNF) in gastrointestinal neoplasms. In phase I studies, complete regressions have been seen with radiotherapy but therapy delivered systemically was limited by significant toxicity. More recently, using an adenoviral vector, locally delivered enhanced intratumoral TNF concentrations of 5-fold have been found with radiotherapy (Gupta *et al.* 2002). This has led to greater growth delay than the vector or radiotherapy alone.

Molecular markers may allow prediction of response to chemotherapy and radiotherapy (Kishi *et al.* 2002) and who will benefit from surgery.

Conclusions

Current studies in oesophageal adenocarcinoma are moving away from chemoradiation, with an emphasis on chemotherapy and surgery. As CRT response rates improve it may be that there will be renewed interest in adenocarcinoma, but more as an alternative to surgery rather than in combination. The role of post-operative radiotherapy and chemoradiotherapy in gastric and oesophageal cancer will need to be re-examined in the light of recent trial results.

Squamous carcinoma will be the subject of studies to improve non-surgical alternatives to resection. Improvements in radiotherapy and systemic therapies should deliver improved local control and treatment of occult metastatic disease. Novel approaches in molecular medicine and with new technology radiotherapy are most likely to produce large step changes in the results from treatment.

References

Al-Sarraf, M., Martz, K. *et al.* (1997). Progress report of combined chemoradiotherapy versus radiotherapy alone in patients with esophageal cancer: an Intergroup study. *Journal of Clinical Oncology* **15**, 277–284.

Apinop, C., Puttisak, P. *et al.* (1994). A prospective study of combined therapy in esophageal cancer. *Hepato-Gastroenterology* **41**, 391–393.

Bains, M. S., Stojadinovic, A. *et al.* (2002). A phase II trial of preoperative combined modality therapy for localized esophageal carcinoma: initial results. *Journal of Thoracic and Cardiovascular Surgery* **124**, 270–277.

Bosset, J. F., Gignoux, M. *et al.* (1997). Chemoradiotherapy followed by surgery compared with surgery alone in squamous-cell cancer of the esophagus. *New England Journal of Medicine* **337**, 161–167.

Burmeister, B. H., Smithers, B. M. *et al.* (2002). Trans Tasman Radiation Oncology Group, Australasian Gastrointestinal Trials Group and Clinical Trials Centre, Sydney, Australia A randomized phase III trial of preoperative chemoradiation followed by surgery (CR-S) versus surgery alone (S) for localized resectable cancer of the esophagus. *Proceedings of the American Society of Clinical Oncology* **21**, 518.

Chan, A. & Wong, A. (1999). Is combined chemotherapy and radiation therapy equally effective as surgical resection in localized esophageal carcinoma. *International Journal of Radiation Oncology, Biology, Physics* **45(2)**, 265–270.

Flamen, P., Lerut, A. *et al.* (2000). Utility of positron emission tomography for the staging of patients with potentially operable esophageal carcinoma. *Journal of Clinical Oncology* **18**, 3202–3210.

Forastiere, A. A., Orringer, M. B. *et al.* (1993). Preoperative chemoradiation followed by transhiatal esophagectomy for carcinoma of the esophagus: final report. *Journal of Clinical Oncology* **11**, 1118–1123.

Gaspar, L. E., Qian, C. *et al.* (1997). A phase I/II study of external beam radiation, brachytherapy and concurrent chemotherapy in localized cancer of the esophagus (RTOG 92-07): preliminary toxicity report. *International Journal of Radiation Oncology, Biology, Physics* **37**, 593–599.

Geh, I. J., Crellin, A. M. *et al.* (2001). A Review of the Role of Preoperative (Neoadjuvant) Chemoradiotherapy in Oesophageal Carcinoma. *British Journal of Surgery* **88**, 338–356.

Gupta, V. K., Park, J. O. *et al.* (2002). Combined gene therapy and ionising radiation is a novel approach to treat human esophageal adenocarcinoma. *Annals of Surgical Oncology* **9(5)**, 500–504.

Kelsen, D. P., Ginsberg, R. *et al.* (1998). Chemotherapy followed by surgery compared with surgery alone for localized esophageal cancer. *New England Journal of Medicine* **339**, 1979–1984.

Kishi, K., Doki, H. *et al.* (2002). Prediction of the response to chemoradiation and prognosis in oesophageal squamous cancer. *British Journal of Surgery* **89**, 597–603.

Lamb, P. J., Immanual, J. *et al.* (2002). Prospective evaluation of bone scintigraphy as a staging investigation for oesophageal carcinoma. *British Journal of Surgery* **89** (Suppl. 1), 26.

Le Prise, E., Etienne, P. L. *et al.* (1994). A randomized study of chemotherapy, radiation therapy, and surgery versus surgery for localized squamous cell carcinoma of the esophagus. *Cancer* **73**, 1779–1784.

Macdonald, J. S., Smalley, S. R. *et al.* (2001). Chemoradiotherapy after surgery compared with surgery alone for adenocarcinoma of the stomach or gastroesophageal junction. *New England Journal of Medicine* **345**, 725–730.

Mandard, A. M., Dalibard, F. *et al.* (1994). Pathologic assessment of tumor regression after preoperative chemoradiotherapy of esophageal carcinoma. *Cancer* **73**, 2680–2686.

Medical Research Council Oesophageal Cancer Working Party (2002). Surgical resection with or without preoperative chemotherapy in oesophageal cancer: a randomised controlled trial. *The Lancet* **359**, 1727–1733.

Minsky, B. D., Neuberg, D. *et al.* (1999). Final report of Intergroup trial 0122 (ECOG PE-289, RTOG 90-12): phase II trial of neoadjuvant chemotherapy plus concurrent chemotherapy and high-dose radiation for squamous cell carcinoma of the esophagus. *International Journal of Radiation Oncology, Biology, Physics* **43**, 517–523.

Miyamoto, T., Yamamoto, H. *et al.* (2003). Carbon ion radiotherapy for stage I non-small cell lung cancer. *Radiotherapy and Oncology* **66**, 127–140.

Nygaard, K., Hagen, S. *et al.* (1992). Pre-operative radiotherapy prolongs survival in operable esophageal carcinoma: a randomized, multicentre study of pre-operative radiotherapy and chemotherapy. The Second Scandinavian Trial in esophageal cancer. *World Journal of Surgery* **16**, 1104–1110.

Sykes, A. J., Burt, P. A. *et al.* (1998). Radical radiotherapy for carcinoma of the oesophagus: an effective alternative to surgery. *Radiotherapy and Oncology* **48**, 15–21.

Urba, S., Orringer, M. *et al.* (2001). Randomised trial of preoperative chemoradiation versus surgery alone in patients with locoregional esophageal carcinoma. *Journal of Clinical Oncology* **19**, 305–313.

Walsh, T. N., Noonan, N. *et al.* (1996). A comparison of multimodal therapy and surgery for esophageal adenocarcinoma. *New England Journal of Medicine* **335**, 462–467.

Wong, R. & Malthaner, R. (2002). Combined chemotherapy and radiotherapy (without surgery) compared with radiotherapy alone in localized carcinoma of the esophagus. *Cochrane Database of Systematic Reviews*.

Xiao, Z. F., Yang, Z. Y. *et al.* (2003). Value of radiotherapy after radical surgery for esophageal carcinoma: A report of 495 patients. *Annals of Thoracic Surgery* **75**, 331–336

Defining the clinical significance of the circumferential margin in gastro-oesophageal cancer

Nicholas Mapstone

Introduction

In the past 20 years there have been few changes in the way that histopathologists have approached upper gastrointestinal cancer resection specimens. Recent improvements in the pathological approach to specimens from elsewhere in the body, increasing treatment options, standardisation and a greater emphasis on quality and completeness in pathological reporting will all increase the quantity and quality of information required from histopathologists in the future.

Circumferential resection margin and other prognostic factors

Traditionally, pathologists have only commented upon involvement by cancer of the proximal and distal resection margins in the oesophagus. This is partly because surgeons have little leeway to increase the width of resection in the oesophagus, and pathologists have not wanted to point out the obvious: that the circumferential resection margin is often involved. There is also a mindset that thinks of a tubular organ as having only proximal and distal margins, not considering that the body of the tube has had to be dissected off adjacent tissues. There is no qualitative difference between a resection margin at either end of a tube and the resection margin surface joining those two ends. One would naturally expect the significance of involvement by cancer of a proximal or distal resection margin (with increased likelihood of local recurrence and worsened prognosis) (Paraf *et al.* 1995; Robeycafferty *et al.* 1991) to be similar to the significance of involvement of the circumferential margin.

There has been wide acceptance of the significance of circumferential resection margin involvement in the rectum for some time. It is associated with a worse prognosis and local recurrence (Adam *et al.* 1994). It is now routinely reported in all rectal and many colonic resection specimens and involvement is often an indication for adjuvant treatment. More proximally margin involvement of pharyngeal tumours has traditionally been documented. Thus involvement of circumferential margins in the hypopharynx (Ho *et al.* 2002) is an independent prognostic factor for overall survival, disease-free survival and nodal recurrence free survival.

With all this circumstantial evidence it would surely be surprising if the oesophagus was the only part of the gastrointestinal tract in which circumferential resection margin involvement was not an important factor.

Circumferential resection margin involvement in the oesophagus has been a peripheral concern in some studies (Mandard *et al.* 1994). Retrospective investigation of a small group of patients found that circumferential resection margin involvement was a significant prognostic factor (Sagar *et al.* 1993). A larger, prospective study (Dexter *et al.* 2002) also found, unsurprisingly, that circumferential resection margin involvement was a significant prognostic factor. They also showed on multivariate analysis that it was the only independently significant prognostic factor in patients with few or no nodal metastases. Thus, in patients with many lymph node metastases, it matters little whether the circumferential resection margin is involved. Circumferential resection margin status only becomes significant in those patients with few or no involved lymph nodes. The odds ratio for the risk of dying from oesophageal cancer was 2.08 when the circumferential resection margin was involved.

An extension of this study with longer follow up (Zafirellis *et al.* 2002) found circumferential resection margin status alone to be significant but only nodal status, vascular invasion and overall R status (R0, resection margins clear macroscopically and microscopically; R1, resection margins clear macroscopically at surgery but later found to be positive microscopically; R2, tumour margins macroscopically involved at surgery) were independent prognostic factors. This 'demotion' of circumferential resection margin status from an independent prognostic factor is initially puzzling. However, by including R status the authors reduced the impact of the circumferential resection margin in multifactorial analysis. Thus the 74 R1 and R2 patients in the study included 66 patients with positive circumferential resection margins and 8 further patients with positive proximal or distal margins. 'R status' is dependent upon circumferential resection margin status.

In another study of 118 patients, circumferential resection margin status was a more important prognostic factor than nodal burden (Saha & Dehn 2001).

Thus there is no doubt that circumferential resection margin status is a significant prognostic factor, and there is some evidence that it is one of the most significant, independent prognostic factors. Margin involvement should always, where possible, be assessed in oesophageal resection specimens. Indeed, it is one of the required parameters in the Royal College of Pathologists Minimum Datasets for the reporting of oesophageal resection specimens (Mapstone 1998). In some hospitals it will not be possible to comment upon the resection margins as the lymph nodes are stripped from the specimen, in theatre, in an attempt to maximise lymph-node yield. This obviously renders the circumferential resection margin inassessable. It is standard Japanese practice for surgeons to dissect lymph nodes from resected specimens, and they have very high lymph-node yields. However, with careful pathological sampling of an oesophageal carcinoma that has been serially sliced, it should be possible to identify all lymph nodes, and allow assessment of resection margins and attain a high lymph-node yield.

Assessment of margin status

There are differing approaches to the pathological assessment of circumferential resection margin status. The Association of Clinical Pathologists broadsheet for oesophageal resection specimens recommends longitudinal slicing of the oesophagus (Ibrahim 2000). This makes the assessment of margin involvement easier in specimens that have been opened for improved fixation. However, this makes it impossible to compare specimen slices with radiological 'slices' from computed tomography (CT) scans. This deprives radiologists of valuable feedback on their predictions of tumour stage and nodal status. Most pathologists slice oesophageal specimens in a horizontal plane in a manner analogous to the dissection of rectal specimens.

There is some discussion of how close a tumour has to be to a circumferential resection margin before the margin is classified as being involved. In the rectum, 1 mm is the traditional cut off point, and it may be this should be extended to 2 mm (Nagtegaal *et al.* 2002). By analogy, 1 mm is the margin used in the oesophagus (Mapstone 1998) but there is no evidence for this. Irrespective of these deliberations, pathologists should document exactly how close tumour approaches to the circumferential resection margin.

Circumferential resection margin status as an indicator of quality of surgery

Resection margin status in the rectum has been suggested as an indicator of the quality of surgery (Birbeck *et al.* 2002; Nagtegaal & van Krieken 2002). A 'good quality' specimen in the rectum has a large and intact capsule of mesorectum surrounding a resected tumour. The anatomy of the mediastinum makes this impossible in oesophageal resection specimens. There are no wide tracts of fat between oesophageal cancers and adjacent, unresectable organs such as the bronchus and heart. Margin status is much more a consequence of the stage of tumour at presentation than the skill of the operator. The number of circumferential resection margin positive oesophageal specimens may be an indicator of the quality of pre-operative staging, but it seems unlikely that it has any relationship to the quality of surgery.

The circumferential resection margin in the stomach

The circumferential resection margin in the stomach is less obvious than that seen in the oesophagus. Tumours of the cardia can potentially involve a circumferential resection margin at the oesophagogastric junction. Indeed, this could be one of the reasons why cardiac tumours have a worse prognosis than tumours in the rest of the stomach. The circumferential resection margin of the rest of the stomach is in the lesser omentum and is extremely difficult to sample with any degree of confidence. Pathologists in the USA are exhorted to determine the status of this circumferential resection margin in their guidelines (Compton & Sobin 1998). Pathologists in the UK have not yet been asked to assess this parameter and there is no evidence that it has any prognostic significance at all.

Standardisation of reporting

The quality of pathological reporting has traditionally been variable (Burroughs *et al.* 1999). The Americans have recommendations (Compton & Sobin 1998), and these are also being published in the UK (Mapstone 1998; Ibrahim 2000). The use of proformas increases the standardisation with which we provide this information (Burroughs *et al.* 1999; Rigby *et al.* 1999). This is crucial for studies and in routine treatment of patients. A recent recommendation by the UICC (Sobin & Wittekind 2002) has changed the pathological criteria for the classification of lymph-node metastases. If these recommendations are followed, many cases that previously would have been N1 would be classified as N0, and vice versa. Thus it is crucial to be specify exactly what is meant by nodal involvement, circumferential resection margin involvement, etc. in any study

The effects of neoadjuvant therapy on pathological reporting

As neoadjuvant treatment is increasingly used and investigated in the treatment of oesophageal cancer, it is crucial that circumferential resection margin status is properly measured. One of the aims of neoadjuvant therapy is to reduce the number of R2 and R1 resections. We will only be able to assess the success of this if circumferential resection margin status is effectively documented. In some studies (Ajani *et al.* 2001; Ancona *et al.* 2001) it is not obvious how R0 status has been assessed. Although there is still disagreement about the relevance of circumferential resection margin status, it is difficult to assume that all resection margins (proximal, distal and circumferential) have been measured without a categorical confirmation of that fact. R0 status in some studies may be completely different from R0 status in other studies.

In some patients the neoadjuvant treatment appears to have had little effect, but in others it is difficult to find any residual viable tumour. An attempt to quantify this effect was first documented in the oesophagus by Mandard *et al.* (1994). They graded tumour regression in five groups: TRG1 (complete regression, absence of residual cancer and fibrosis extending throughout the different layers of the esophageal wall); TRG2 (rare residual cancer cells scattered throughout the fibrosis); TRG 3 (an increase in the number of residual cancer cells but fibrosis still predominates); TRG4 (residual cancer outgrowing fibrosis); and TRG5 (absence of regressive changes). These assessments are essentially subjective and there are no data available about the degree of inter- and intraobserver variation encountered when using them. Darnton *et al* (1993) used the proportion of tumour to stroma to assess the effect of chemotherapy on squamous cell carcinoma.

Some pathologists routinely take three blocks of tissue from a tumour, which may well sample only 10% of the tumour. Other pathologists might attempt to sample all of a neoadjuvantly treated tumour with, for example, 10 blocks of tissue. Complete regression as assessed by the latter is obviously a much more robust concept than complete regression documented by the former. Thus there should be guidance of how much of a tumour should be sampled before a diagnosis of complete regression should be made. Sometimes a tumour, which has shrunk after chemoradiotherapy, may leave behind mucin 'pools' with no obviously viable tumour cells in them. A mucin pool within lymph nodes strongly suggests that tumour was present in that node before treatment (Weese *et al.* 2000). Any study of neoadjuvant treatment should specify whether these mucin pools are treated as the presence of viable tumour (usually not) and how hard pathologists should look for viable cells within these mucin pools. Thus, should immunohistochemistry for cytokeratins be used to identify epithelial cells within these mucin pools?

Conclusion

In summary there are few excuses for any pathologist not to document involvement of the circumferential resection margin in oesophageal (but not gastric) carcinoma resection specimens. This information will provide some prognostic information but little evidence about the quality of surgery. It will, however, be crucial to have good-quality standardised information about the circumferential resection margin status and tumour regression in any study concerned with new treatment modalities, either for assessing treatment effectiveness or its impact on prognosis.

References

Adam, I. J., Mohamdee, M. O. Martin, I. G. *et al.* (1994). Role of circumferential margin involvement in the local recurrence of rectal cancer. *The Lancet* **344**, 707–711.

Ajani, J. A., Komaki, R. Putnam, J. B. *et al.* (2001). A three-step strategy of induction chemotherapy then chemoradiation followed by surgery in patients with potentially resectable carcinoma of the esophagus or gastroesophageal junction. *Cancer* **92**, 279–286.

Ancona, E., Ruol, A. Santi, S. *et al.* (2001). Only pathologic complete response to neoadjuvant chemotherapy improves significantly the long term survival of patients with resectable esophageal squamous cell carcinoma: final report of a randomized, controlled trial of preoperative chemotherapy versus surgery alone. *Cancer* **91**, 2165–2174.

Birbeck, K. F., Macklin, C. P., Tiffin, N. J. *et al.* (2002). Rates of circumferential resection margin involvement vary between surgeons and predict outcomes in rectal cancer surgery. *Annals of Surgery* **235**, 449–457

Burroughs, S. H., Biffin, A. H., Pye, J. K. & Williams, G. T. (1999). Oesophageal and gastric cancer pathology reporting: a regional audit. *Journal of Clinical Pathology* **52**, 435–439.

Compton, C. & Sobin, L. H. (1998). Protocol for the examination of specimens removed from patients with gastric carcinoma: a basis for checklists. Members of the Cancer Committee, College of American Pathologists, and the Task Force for Protocols on the Examination of Specimens from Patients with Gastric Cancer. *Archives of Pathology and Laboratory Medicine* **122**, 9–14.

Darnton, S. J., Allen, S. M., Edwards, C. W. & Matthews, H. R. (1993). Histopathological findings in oesophageal carcinoma with and without preoperative chemotherapy. *Journal of Clinical Pathology* **46**, 51–55.

Dexter, F., Lubarsky, D. A. & Blake, J. T. (2002). Sampling error can significantly affect measured hospital financial performance of surgeons and resulting operating room time allocations. *Anesthesia and Analgesia* **95**, 184–188.

Ho, C. M., Ng, W. F., Lam, K. H. *et al.* (2002). Radial clearance in resection of hypopharyngeal cancer: an independent prognostic factor. *Head and Neck* **24**, 181–190.

Ibrahim, N. (2000). Guidelines for handling oesophageal biopsies and resection specimens and their reporting. *Journal of Clinical Pathology* **53**, 89–94.

Mandard, A. M., Dalibard, F. Mandard, J. C. *et al.* (1994). Pathologic assessment of tumor regression after preoperative chemoradiotherapy of esophageal carcinoma. Clinicopathologic correlations. *Cancer* **73**, 2680–2686.

Mapstone, N. P. (1998). Standards and Minimum Datasets for Reporting Common Cancers: Minimum dataset for oesophageal cancer histopathology reports. London: The Royal College of Pathologists.

Nagtegaal, I. D., Marijnen, C. A., Kranenbarg, E. K. *et al.* (2002). Circumferential margin involvement is still an important predictor of local recurrence in rectal carcinoma: not one millimeter but two millimeters is the limit. *American Journal of Surgical Pathology* **26**, 350–357.

Nagtegaal, I. D. & van Krieken, J. H. (2002). The role of pathologists in the quality control of diagnosis and treatment of rectal cancer–an overview. *European Journal of Cancer* **38**, 964–972.

Paraf, F., Flejou, J. F., Pignon, J. P. *et al.* (1995). Surgical pathology of adenocarcinoma arising in Barretts-esophagus – analysis of 67 cases. *American Journal of Surgical Pathology* **19**, 183–191.

Rigby, K., Brown, S. R., Lakin, G. *et al.* (1999). The use of a proforma improves colorectal cancer pathology reporting. *Annals of the Royal College of Surgeons of England* **81**, 401–403.

Robeycafferty, S. S., Elnaggar, A. K. Sahin, A. A. *et al.* (1991). Prognostic factors in esophageal squamous carcinoma – a study of histologic features, blood-group expression, and DNA ploidy. *American Journal of Clinical Pathology* **95**, 844–849.

Sagar, P. M., Johnston, D., McMahon, M. J. *et al.* (1993). Significance of circumferential resection margin involvement after oesophagectomy for cancer. *British Journal of Surgery* **80**, 1386–1388.

Saha, S. & Dehn, T. C. (2001). Ratio of invaded to removed lymph nodes as a prognostic factor in adenocarcinoma of the distal esophagus and esophagogastric junction. *Diseases of the Esophagus* **14**, 32–36.

Sobin, L. & Wittekind, C. (eds) (2002). *TNM classification of malignant tumours.* New York: John Wiley.

Weese, J. L., Harbison, S. P., Stiller, G. D. *et al.* (2000). Neoadjuvant chemotherapy, radical resection with intraoperative radiation therapy (IORT): improved treatment for gastric adenocarcinoma. *Surgery* **128**, 564–571.

Zafirellis, K., Dolan, K., Fountoulakis, A. *et al.* (2002). Multivariate analysis of clinical, operative and pathologic features of esophageal cancer: who needs adjuvant therapy? *Diseases of the Esophagus* **15**, 155–159.

Chapter 7

The adjuvant treatment of gastric cancer

Martin Hogg, Vincent Khoo, Ian Welch and Mark Saunders

Introduction

For those who are fit enough for surgery, resection is the treatment of choice for patients with potentially curable gastric carcinoma. The extent of disease at presentation determines resectability, and also long-term survival. Unfortunately, in the West, most patients present at an advanced stage and therefore curative resection rates are low (Allum *et al.* 1989; Akoh & Macintyre 1992; Cuschieri *et al.* 1996). Any measures that facilitate detection of gastric carcinoma at an early stage should lead to improved resectability rates and improved post-operative survival (Sue-Ling *et al.* 1993; Hallissey *et al.* 1990).

Until recently there was no proven role for adjuvant chemotherapy, radiotherapy or synchronous chemo-radiotherapy. However, two meta-analyses and several small adjuvant chemotherapy studies have been published with encouraging results. There is also a large randomised study showing a significant survival benefit with post-operative adjuvant chemo-radiotherapy. However, there is considerable debate as to the optimal surgical management for this group of patients and in particular, the extent of lymph node dissection. This chapter is devoted to reviewing and discussing the overall management of adjuvant therapy for gastric cancer.

Surgery for gastric cancer

Gastric carcinoma tends to behave as a loco-regional disease with distant metastases occurring later in a significant proportion of patients. Studies from Japan indicate that patients with gastric carcinoma can be cured, even in the presence of loco-regional lymph node metastases if they undergo a D2 or 'systematic' lymphadenectomy (Table 7.1). This involves wide excision of the gastric primary together with the greater omentum and the first two tiers of lymph nodes that drain the area of the stomach affected by the carcinoma. An 'extended' or D3 lymphadenectomy involves resection of lymph nodes beyond the second tier of nodes. Resection of only the first tier of nodes is a D1 or 'limited' lymphadenectomy. Until recently, this has traditionally been the level of resection performed by most surgeons in the West. The Japanese rules for gastric surgery suggest that resection is likely to afford an absolute cure if all evidence of carcinoma is resected locally and if at least one tier of nodes beyond those affected with metastases is resected (for example a D2 lymphadenectomy for carcinoma where there is either no nodal involvement or if only the first tier of nodes are involved (Maruyama *et al.* 1989)).

Table 7.1 Surgery for gastric cancer

Type of surgery	Lymphadenectomy for gastric carcinoma
D0	Gastric resection and incomplete resection of local lymph nodes
D1	Gastric resection with removal of lymph nodes within 3.0cm of the tumour
D2	Gastric resection with removal of lymph nodes within 3.0cm of the tumour and the nodes along the main arteries supplying the stomach
D3	A more radical *en bloc* resection including removal of lymph nodes outside the normal lymphatic pathways from the stomach. Involved in advanced stages or by retrograde lymphatic flare due to blockage of normal pathways. N.B. The tiers of lymph nodes are different for each part of the stomach

Comparison of post-operative survival rates for patients with equivalent stage carcinoma shows significantly poorer results in Western series compared with those from Japan (Akoh & Macintyre 1992). However, caution is needed in interpreting these results to avoid the 'stage migration' effect that can result from the more accurate pathological staging of disease (Table 7.2) by the more extensive 'Japanese-type' lymph node resection. The differences therefore, may not be solely attributable to the surgery alone. Compared with Japan, at least two European units have shown similar post-operative survival rates after D2 gastrectomy and lymphadenectomy, particularly for early-stage disease (Siewert *et al.* 1993; Sue-Ling *et al.* 1993). It is possible that the benefit of a D2 resection is confined mainly to stage II and IIIa disease (Siewert *et al.* 1996) (Table 7.3). Furthermore, it is possible that a proportion of patients with second-tier nodal involvement are also cured by D2 lymphadenectomy (Maruyama *et al.* 1989, Seto *et al.* 1997).

Table 7.2 TNM classification of gastric carcinoma

Tis* T1 (early gastric cancer) T2 T3 T4	Tumour invades: Lamina propria, submucosa Muscularis propria, subserosa Serosa Adjacent structures
N1;	1–6 nodes involved;
N2;	7–15 nodes involved;
N3	>15 nodes involved
M1	Distant metastasis present
M0	No distant metastases
N0	No lymph nodes involved

*Carcinoma *in situ*: intraepithelial tumour without invasion of lamina propria.

Table 7.3 Stage grouping for gastric carcinoma

Stage 0 Stage 1A	Tis T1 T1 T2	N0 N0 N1	M0 M0 M0
Stage 1B		N0	M0
Stage II	T1 T2 T3	N2 N1 N0	M0 M0 M0
Stage IIIA	T2 T3 T4	N2 N1 N0	M0 M0 M0
Stage IIIB	T3	N2	M0
Stage IV	T4 T1, T2, T3 Any T	N1, N2, N3 N3 Any N	M0 M0 M1

Two multi-centre trials from Europe have failed to demonstrate a survival benefit favouring D2 over D1 surgery for gastric carcinoma (Cuschieri *et al.* 1999; Bonenkamp *et al.* 1999). In fact, the mortality after surgery was higher for the D2 resection groups in both trials. This may be partly due to the splenectomy and distal pancreatectomy, which was performed in addition to the D2 lymph node dissection in several patients. Despite these findings, the International Gastric Cancer Association Consensus (1997) favoured a D2 lymphadenectomy for patients with curable gastric cancer.

The addition of splenectomy to surgical resection of gastric carcinoma appears to adversely affect prognosis (Griffith *et al.* 1995; Wanebo *et al.* 1997). Splenectomy is sometimes performed because of concern that the splenic hilar nodes may contain metastatic carcinoma. This is a distinct possibility in more advanced and surgically incurable carcinoma but is present in fewer than 1% of patients with curable carcinoma of the antrum and less than 10% of those with carcinoma of the middle-third of the stomach (Okajama & Isozaki 1995). Resection of the splenic hilar nodes without splenectomy is technically feasible and is performed in Japan but is still under investigation in the West.

The addition of distal pancreatectomy to surgical resection of gastric carcinoma may be performed to allow resection of lymph nodes along the length of the splenic artery. It also forms part of the surgery for otherwise potentially resectable T4 tumours of the stomach with direct posterior invasion into the pancreas itself. Distal pancreatectomy appears to be associated with significant morbidity and possibly a worse prognosis, than for patients who do not undergo pancreatectomy. However, other factors may also contribute to these observations (Cuschieri *et al.* 1999). Similar to the situation with splenic hilar nodes, excision of splenic artery nodes without pancreatectomy is also feasible and is under assessment (Maruyama *et al.* 1995).

There are guidelines for the extent of gastric resection according to the site and size of the carcinoma. These guidelines also provide the acceptable margins of macroscopic clearance required (Japanese Research Society for Gastric Cancer 1995). For a diffuse tumour with sub-mucosal infiltration and for infiltrative tumours where there is less than 5 cm clearance proximally from the cardia, a total gastrectomy is indicated. A sub-total gastrectomy is appropriate for a well-circumscribed tumour (T1, T2) if the proximal margin of the tumour is more than 2 cm distal to the cardia. For type II and III oesophago-gastric junction tumours (Table 7.4), a total gastrectomy with lymphadenectomy may again be considered. This should also include resection of the distal oesophagus with the proximal resection margin sited at least 5 cm above the proximal extent of the macroscopic tumour. *En bloc* resection of pancreas, diaphragm or left lobe of liver may be considered where there is direct tethering or invasion by tumour provided that the patient is considered fit enough for this magnitude of surgery and that resection still has the aim of potential cure.

Table 7.4 Classification of junctional tumours

Oesophago-gastric junctional tumours	Carcinoma involves:
Type I	Distal oesophagus
Type II	Cardia
Type III	Proximal stomach

In several Japanese patients with early gastric carcinoma, less extensive gastric resections are now being performed, both as open or laparoscopic surgery and even via the gastroscope. However, for similar, apparently early tumours in Western patients, there appears to be a significant incidence of nodal metastases at the time of surgery. Hence, this type of limited resection may not be appropriate for this cohort of patients in the West (Hayes *et al.* 1996).

In the palliative setting where disease is not amenable to cure, one may consider surgery for symptom control. For example, distal gastrectomy or gastro-enterostomy for malignant gastric outlet obstruction or limited resection for a lesion which has bled significantly. Endoscopic or radiological placement of expandable metal stents across the distal stomach and pylorus to palliate outlet obstruction is practised in some centres, but widespread experience so far in the West is limited (Uno *et al.* 1997).

The mortality and morbidity after surgery for gastric carcinoma is influenced by many factors. Palliative operations are associated with higher mortality than potentially curative procedures. Total gastrectomy has twice the expected mortality of sub-total gastrectomy. Surgeons performing nine or more resections per year appear to have a lower operative mortality than those performing less than this number (Allum *et al.* 1989). Furthermore, specialist units may have post-operative mortality rates of less than 5%. These observations have added weight to the argument that there may be an advantage in concentrating surgical and multi-disciplinary expertise in specialist centres (Siewert *et al.* 1993; Sue-Ling *et al.* 1993), In the West, the post-operative mortality for D2 resection is higher than that for D1 resection although there are several potential confounding factors that may contribute to this difference. In addition, there is some evidence of a learning curve for D2 surgery; hence, increased experience and expertise may reduce morbidity and mortality in the future (Parikh *et al.* 1996).

Early adjuvant chemotherapy and radiotherapy trials

Initial adjuvant chemotherapy and radiotherapy trials for gastric cancer revealed conflicting results. Between 1978 and 1989, Zhang *et al.* (1998) randomised 370 patients to surgery or surgery plus pre-operative radiotherapy to 40 Gy in 20 fractions over 4 weeks using a parallel-opposed pair of fields. Radiotherapy was delivered 2–4 weeks before surgery. The survival curves of the two groups diverged significantly early on and remained apart ($p = 0.0094$). However, the 5-year survival rates were lower than other reports in the literature, being 30% in the combined group and 20% in the surgery alone group.

In 1969, Moertel *et al.* randomised 62 patients to surgery alone or post-operative chemo-radiotherapy (37.5 Gy in 4–5 weeks with concomitant 5-fluorouracil (5-FU) (15 mg/kg/day × 3 by i.v. bolus)). A significant survival advantage was demonstrated for the combined modality arm. However, this study has to be interpreted with some caution. Informed consent was only gained from those patients who received chemo-radiotherapy and 10 of the 39 patients randomised to the intervention arm refused treatment and were subsequently assigned to the observational arm.

A meta-analysis was performed of 11 post-operative adjuvant chemotherapy trials, published between 1982 and 1991 (Hermans *et al.* 1993). A total of 2,096 patients were included in this study and patients received mainly 5-FU-based chemotherapy regimens. A survival benefit was not shown and therefore, in the early 1990s, adjuvant chemotherapy was not recommended after curative resection of a stomach cancer.

The second British Stomach Cancer Group trial of adjuvant radiotherapy or chemotherapy in resectable gastric cancer demonstrated the British experience (Hallissey *et al.* 1994). This trial considered 436 patients prospectively randomised to surgery alone (145), surgery and radiotherapy (153) and surgery and combination chemotherapy (138) (FAM: fluorouracil 600 mg/m^2, adriamycin 30 mg/m^2, mitomycin 4 mg/m^2; 3 weekly for eight cycles). Radiotherapy was given as parallel-opposed pair of fields to a dose of 45 Gy in 25 fractions over 5 weeks. A 5 Gy boost to a smaller field was optional. Surgeons recorded disease according to the Japanese Research Society for Gastric Cancer (JRSGC). Loco-regional failure as a component of initial failure was documented in 39 of the 145 patients in the surgery only arm (27%), 26 of the 138 patients in the FAM group (19%) and in only 15 of the 153 patients that received post-operative radiotherapy (10%; log-rank $p < 0.01$). However, a survival advantage was not found. There were several perceived problems with this study. Of the patients randomised into this study, 144 (33%) had residual disease while a further 78 patients (18%) had positive margins. Such patients would not normally be eligible for adjuvant trials. Formal quality assurance evaluation of the radiotherapy fields was also not reported and approximately a third of those patients irradiated, received <40.5 Gy. Nonetheless, a significant reduction in local failure was found in this group of patients.

Later adjuvant chemotherapy trials

Two recent meta-analyses suggest that adjuvant chemotherapy may be beneficial. The first included a total of 1255 patients in 13 randomised studies between 1980 and 1996 (Earle & Maroun 1999). An odds ratio for death in the treated group of 0.80 (95% confidence interval (CI) 0.66–0.97) corresponding to a relative risk of 0.94 (95% CI 0.89–1.00) was demonstrated. A trend for a larger effect was seen in the node positive sub-group. Mari et $al.$ (2000) considered 3,658 cases from 20 randomised controlled trials published between 1983 and 1999. 5-Fluorouracil was used in combination with other cytotoxic agents in all but three of trials included in this meta-analysis. They showed that chemotherapy reduced the risk of death by 18% (hazard ratio of 0.82, 95% CI 0.75–0.89, $p < 0.001$). They concluded that chemotherapy does provide a small survival benefit; however, given the limitations of a meta-analysis, they recommended that suitable patients should still be entered into clinical trials.

Two further studies have recently been published whereby patients were randomised to receive adjuvant chemotherapy or no further therapy following curative resection of a gastric cancer. Neri et $al.$ (2001) randomised 137 lymph-node-positive patients to epidoxorubicin (75 mg/m^2 day 1), leucovorin (200 mg/m^2 day 1–3) and 5-FU (450 mg/m^2 day 1–3) 3 weekly for eight cycles after curative resection. With a median follow up of 5 years, the median overall survival was 18 months for controls and 31 months for the treatment arm. The 5-year overall survival was 13% and 30%, respectively ($p < 0.001$). The estimated hazard ratio for mortality of the control versus treatment arm was 1.96 (95% CI 1.32–2.92). Cirera et $al.$ (1999) randomised 148 patients after curative resection of stage III gastric cancer to no further treatment or mitomycin-C and oral tegafur for 3 months. Median survival was 29 months for the control group and 74 months for the treatment group ($p = 0.04$). Disease-free survival was 22 versus 63 months, respectively, after median follow-up of 37 months ($p = 0.01$). Two- and five-year overall survival was 58% and 36% for the control group, and 72% and 56% for the treatment group. Estimated hazard ratio for mortality in the treatment group versus control was 0.60 (95% CI 0.39–0.93). There was a larger percentage of patients with affected nodes in the control group (93%) compared with the treatment group (80%); however, these differences did not reach statistical significance ($p = 0.07$).

In summary therefore, two meta-analyses and two small randomised studies have suggested that adjuvant chemotherapy may be beneficial. However, the exact type of chemotherapy remains undecided, although most of the regimens contained a fluoropyrimidine. The "MAGIC" study (MRC Adjuvant Gastric Infusional Chemotherapy) compared three cycles of ECF chemotherapy (epirubicin, cisplatin, infusional 5-FU) before and immediately after surgery (CSC), to surgery (S) alone for patients with resectable gastric cancer (Cunningham *et al.* 2003). Five hundred and three patients were randomised into this study over 8 years between 1994 and 2002. Resection was considered curative in 79% of patients receiving the combined therapy compared with 69% of patients who received surgery alone ($p = 0.02$). The number of 'open and close' procedures was reduced by more than 50% if chemotherapy was given before surgery (11% to 5%). Post-operative complications were similar (CSC 47%, S 45%) as were deaths within 30 days (CSC 6%, S 6%). For those patients who received pre-operative chemotherapy, more of the resected tumours were smaller and of an earlier stage (Maximum diameter 3 cm (range 2–6 cm) for CSC patients and 5cm (range 3–8 cm) for surgery only patients ($p < 0.001$); T1/T2: 51% versus 36% ($p = 0.01$)). Progression-free survival was significantly better in the CSC arm ($p = 0.002$) and there was a trend towards an improved overall survival at 2 years in the cohort of patients that received chemotherapy (48% versus 40%; $p = 0.06$).

Adjuvant chemoradiotherapy

Macdonald *et al.* (2001) randomised 556 patients with curatively resected adenocarcinoma of the stomach or gastro-oesophageal junction to no further treatment or adjuvant chemo-radiotherapy, 20–40 days after surgery. The median age was 59 (range 23–80) for the surgical group, and 60 years (range 25–87) for the surgery plus chemo-radiotherapy group. Adjuvant treatment consisted of an initial cycle of 5-FU (425 mg/m^2) and leucovorin (20 mg/m^2) for five consecutive days, one month before chemoradiotherapy. The 5-FU dose was reduced to 400 mg/m^2 during the radiotherapy and was given for the first four days and final three days of treatment. Radiotherapy was delivered as a parallel-opposed pair to a dose of 45 Gy, using at least 4 MV photons, to the midline, in 25 fractions over 5 weeks (Figure 7.1). The clinical target volume included the tumour bed, 2 cm beyond the proximal and distal resection margins and regional nodes. The tumour bed was defined with information from the operation, pre-operative CT scanning, and barium roentography (Smalley *et al.* 2001). An example of a typical radiotherapy treatment volume using this protocol from a patient treated at the Christie Hospital, Manchester, is depicted in Figure 7.2.

If the lesion was T3 the left hemi-diaphragm was included in the treatment fields. Lymph nodes were defined using the guidelines of the JRSGC. Perigastric, coeliac, local para-aortic, splenic, hepato-duodenal or hepatic portal, and pancreato-duodenal lymph nodes were included in the fields. Gastro-oesophageal tumour fields included para-cardial and para-oesophageal but excluded pancreato-duodenal lymph nodes. If it was necessary to spare the left kidney, the splenic nodes were excluded. Less than

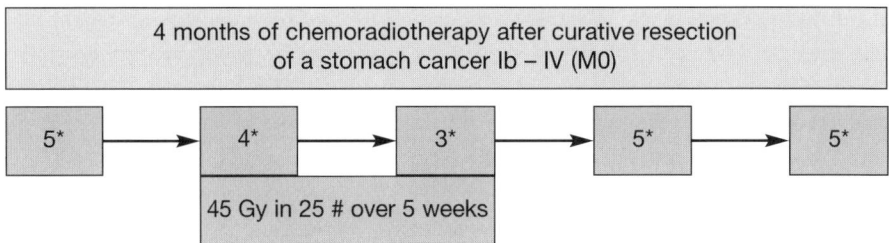

*3–5 day 5-FU/leucovorin chemotherapy. 5-FU 425 mg/m^2/day without radiotherapy and 400 mg/m^2/day with radiotherapy given for 3–5 consecutive days as described above (leucovorin 20 mg/m^2/day).

Figure 7.1 Treatment schema for Macdonald *et al.* (2001) trial.

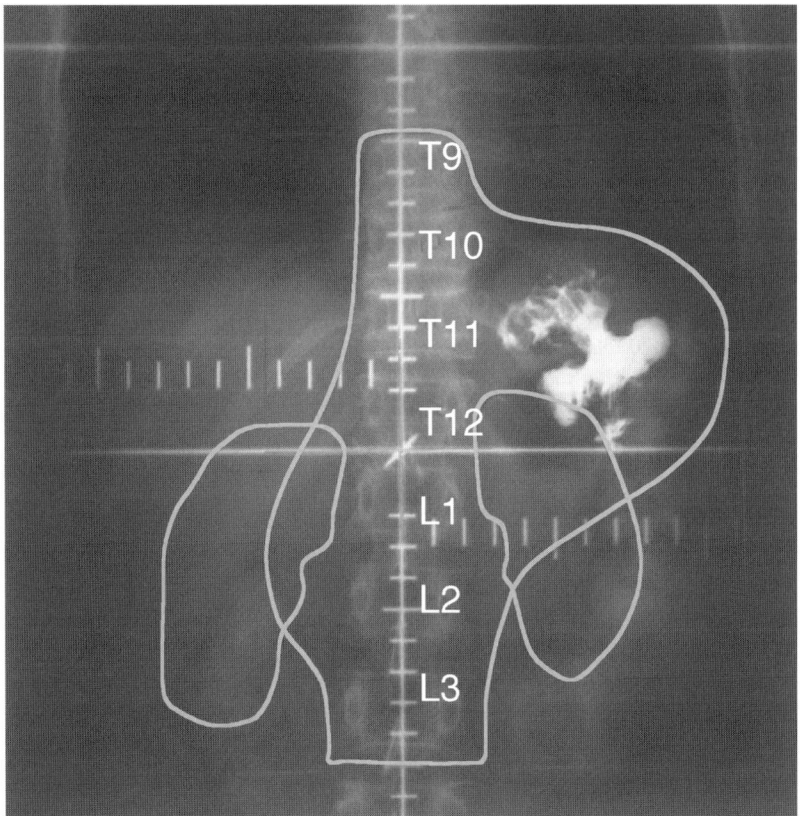

Figure 7.2 An example of typical radiotherapy treatment volume. The planning target volume and position of the kidneys are marked on the film.

60% of the hepatic volume was to be exposed to more than 30 Gy, and no portion of the heart representing 30% of the cardiac volume received more than 40 Gy. In the trial, all plans were reviewed before implementation and 35% contained 'major or minor deviations'. Most were corrected before radiotherapy; however, a quality-assurance review after the treatment had been delivered demonstrated that 6.5% of cases still exhibited major deviations from the treatment plans.

Of those 281 randomised to receive adjuvant treatment, only 64% completed the schedule as planned. Of the remainder, 17% stopped early because of toxic effects, 8% declined further treatment, while 5% progressed during treatment and 4% stopped for other reasons. Toxicity of grade 3 or higher was noted as follows: haematological (commonly leucopaenia) 54%; gastro-intestinal (nausea, vomiting and diarrhoea) 33%; influenza-like 9%; infection 3%; neurological 4%; cardiovascular 4%; pain 3%; metabolic 2%; hepatic 1%; lung related 1%; death 1% (three patients).

With a median follow-up of 5 years, the median survival was 27 months in the control group and 36 months in the treatment group. Three-year survival was 41% in the control group and 51% in the treatment group, with a hazard ratio for death in the control group relative to the chemo-radiotherapy group of 1.35 (95% CI 1.09–1.66; p = 0.005). In summary, the authors suggest that this form of adjuvant chemo-radiotherapy should be considered for appropriate patients that have had a curative resection of their gastric carcinoma.

However, several criticisms have been levelled at it. Perhaps the most serious was that the trial was only positive because of the relatively poor outcome in the surgery alone arm (41% 3-year survival) and that the surgery undertaken was inadequate. In the Macdonald study a D2 dissection was recommended but this occurred in only 10% of patients, with 36% having a D1 dissection and 54% of the 552 patients receiving a D0 dissection. Even though they were unable to detect a difference in relapse-free and overall survival according to the extent of surgery, the high proportion of D0 resections was considered unacceptable by some authors (Atkins 2002; Berney and Merrett 2002). The outcome for patients in the Dutch Gastric Cancer Group study is certainly better, with a 5-year survival of 47% after D1 resection and 45% after D2 resection (Bonenkamp *et al.* 1999). However, the 85% of patients in the MacDonald study had positive nodes compared with only 55% in the Dutch study. There were also more T3 tumours in the MacDonald cohort of patients. In support of the MacDonald study, Kelsen (2000) argued that the 3-year survival of the surgery only arm is comparable to the larger American experience in the American College of Surgeons Patient Care Study (Wanebo *et al.* 1993). In this review, 3,044 patients had a curative resection giving a 3-year survival of 42%. In the MacDonald study, the patients were identified post-operatively and were stratified according to the local extent (T-stage) and nodal status of the tumour. Abraham *et al.* (2002) suggested that randomisation should take place pre-operatively and agreed with others that the type of surgery should have been more uniform. They also queried whether this form of chemoradiotherapy, with significant toxicity and poor compliance, was worth suffering for a 9-month median survival benefit.

However, despite these criticisms, this large prospective multicentre randomised study appears well constructed and includes only patients who had a complete resection with negative margins. There was a good attempt at quality assurance of the radiotherapy with review of the proposed treatment by a single radiation oncologist and correction of any deviations before starting therapy. The authors also quite rightly stated that the radiation oncologist should be familiar with this technique and that good support during the therapy was essential. They concluded that this treatment should be considered for high-risk patients after a curative resection of a gastric or gastro-oesophageal tumour.

An audit of our local experience using the same protocol described above, revealed 17 patients treated by a single radiation oncologist between April 2000 and October 2002. All patients had had a curative resection and all patients had negative margins. All patients had locally advanced tumours, with 71% having positive lymph nodes. In this cohort, all but two patients received the planned dose of radiotherapy (Figure 7.2). Most patients (65%) received all of the concurrent chemotherapy; however, only seven patients completed all five cycles of chemotherapy. The final two cycles of chemotherapy, given after the radiotherapy had been completed, were the hardest for patients to cope with. At this point, patients need to concentrate on improving their nutritional status, which is sometimes difficult when they are also receiving further chemotherapy. Grade 3 toxicity was noted in seven patients (41%), while one of these patients also developed grade 4 neutropaenia. The predominant problems were neutropaenia, nausea, weight-loss and lethargy. Currently, there is inadequate follow-up for late toxicity data; however, there are no obvious complications so far. Eleven patients were alive and well at their last follow-up appointment, and there were no treatment-related deaths. In our experience this treatment is feasible, although it is important to select patients of good performance status and we agree with MacDonald *et al.* (2001) that good support (both nutritional and psychological) is essential.

Conclusion

Adjuvant treatment is now an option to consider for patients who have had a curative resection of a gastric cancer. For years, there was no adjuvant therapy that was proven to be useful. Two meta-analyses have shown that adjuvant chemotherapy of some sort provides a significant increase in overall survival (Earle & Maroun 1999; Mari *et al.* 2000). Two recent post-operative adjuvant chemotherapy studies, based on fluorinated pyrimidines, have also shown a significant survival advantage when this therapy is given after a gastric cancer has been curatively resected (Cirera *et al.* 1999; Neri *et al.* 2001).

Chemoradiotherapy together with adjuvant 5-FU and folinic acid has been shown to provide a significant survival advantage by MacDonald *et al.* (2001). This well-constructed randomised study does have its faults, mainly related to the completeness of the surgery. However, it could provide the basis for future studies using improved radiotherapy techniques, together with other chemotherapeutic agents such as cisplatin and newer ones including capecitabine and irinotecan. Ideally it would be appropriate to treat such patients as part of a well-constructed clinical trial. With this ideal in mind, a phase I/II chemoradiotherapy study was started last year at The Netherlands Cancer Institute (NKI) and Christie Hospital in Manchester (UK). Intravenous 5-FU has been replaced with capecitabine and the radiotherapy planning technique has been modified and improved. It is hoped that this trial will be used as a template for a follow-on study to MAGIC in the UK. The aim would be to use the information gained from this trial (Cunningham *et al.* 2003) and the North American study (MacDonald *et al.* 2001), to create a National randomised trial incorporating efficacious treatment with good surgical, pathological and radiotherapy quality control. Whatever the treatment chosen or trial formulated, it must be given by a team dedicated and experienced in the treatment of this malignancy. Good cooperation between the gastroenterologist, surgeon, pathologist, radiologist and oncologist is essential.

References

Abraham, I., Dhar, P. & Praseedom, R. K. (2002). Adjuvant chemo-radiotherapy for gastric cancer. *New England Journal of Medicine* **346**, 210–211.

Allum, W. H., Powell. D. J. & McConkey. C. C. *et al.* (1989). Gastric cancer: a 25 year review. *British Journal of Surgery* **76**, 535–540.

Akoh, J. A. & Macintyre, I. M. C. (1992). Improving survival in gastric cancer: a review of 5-year survival rates in English language publications from 1970. *British Journal of Surgery* **79**, 293–299.

Atkins, C. D. (2002). Adjuvant chemo-radiotherapy for gastric cancer. *New England Journal of Medicine* **346**, 210–211.

Berney, C. R. & Merrett, N. D. (2002). Adjuvant chemo-radiotherapy for gastric cancer. *New England Journal of Medicine* **346** (3), 210–211.

Bonenkamp, J. J., Hermans, J., Sasako, M. *et al.* (1999). Extended lymph node dissection for gastric cancer. Dutch gastric cancer group. *New England Journal of Medicine* **340**, 908–914.

Ciera, L., Balil, A., Batiste-Alentorn, E. *et al.* (1999). Randomised clinical trial of adjuvant mitomycin plus tegafur in patients with resected stage 111 gastric cancer. *Journal of Clinical Oncology* **17**, 3810–3815.

Cunningham, D., Allum, W. & Weedon, S. (2003). Perioperative chemotherapy in operable gastric and lower oesophageal cancer: a randomised, controlled trial of the NCRI Upper GI Clinical Studies Group (the MAGIC trial, ISRCTN 93793971. *European Journal of Cancer* **39**(Suppl. 5), SI8.

Cuschieri, A., Fayers, P., Fielding, J. *et al.* (1996). Postoperative morbidity and mortality after D1 and D2 resections for gastric cancer: preliminary results of the MRC randomised controlled surgical trial. *The Lancet* **347**, 995–999.

Cuschieri, A., Weeden, S., Fielding, J. *et al*. (1999). Patient survival after D1 and D2 resections for gastric cancer: long term results of the MRC randomised surgical trial. Surgical Co-operative group. *British Journal of Cancer* **79**, 1522–1530.

Earle, C. C. & Marounm, J. A. (1999). Adjuvant chemotherapy after curative resection for gastric cancer in Non-Asian patients: Revisiting a Meta-analysis of randomised trials. *European Journal of Cancer* **35**, 1059–1064.

Griffith, J. P., Sue-Ling, H., Johnston, D. *et al.* (1995). Preservation of the spleen improves survival after radical surgery for gastric cancer. *Gut* **36**, 684–690.

Hallissey, M. T., Allum, W. H., Jewkes, A. J. *et al.* (1990). Early detection of gastric cancer. *British Medical Journal* **301**, 513–515.

Hallissey, M. T., Dunn, J. A., Ward, L. C. & Allum, W. H. (1994). For the British Stomach Cancer Group. The second British Stomach Cancer Group trial of adjuvant radiotherapy or chemotherapy in resectable gastric cancer: five-year follow-up. *The Lancet* **343**, 1309–1312.

Hayes, N., Karat, D. & Scott, D. J. *et al.* (1996). Radical lymphadenectomy in the management of early gastric cancer. *British Journal of Surgery* **83**, 1421–1423.

Hermans, J., Bonenkamp, J. J., Boon, M. C. *et al.* (1993). Adjuvant therapy after curative resection for gastric cancer: meta-analysis of randomised trials. *Journal of Clinical Oncology* **11**, 1441–1447.

Japanese Research Society for Gastric Cancer (1995). *Japanese classification of gastric cancer*, 1st English edition. Tokyo: Ilanetiara.

Kelsen, D. P. (2000). Post-operative adjuvant chemoradiation therapy for patients with resected gastric cancer: Intergroup 116. *Journal of Clinical Oncology* **18**, 32–34.

MacDonald, J. S. Smalley, S. R., Benedetti, J. *et al.* (2001). Chemo-radiotherapy after surgery compared with surgery alone for adenocarcinoma of the stomach or gastro-oesophageal junction. *New England Journal of Medicine* **345**, 725–730.

Mari, E., Floriani, I., Tinazzi, A. *et al.* (2000). Efficacy adjuvant chemotherapy after curative resection for gastric cancer: a meta-analysis of published randomised trials. *Annals of Oncology* **11**, 837–843.

Maruyama, K., Gunven, P., Okabayashi, K. *et al.* (1989). Lymph node metastases of gastric cancer. General pattern in 1931 patients. *Annals of Surgery* **210**, 596–602.

Maruyama, K., Sasako, M., Kinoshita, T. *et al.* (1995). Pancreas-preserving total gastrectomy for proximal gastric cancer. *World Journal of Surgery* **19**, 532–536.

Moertel, C. G., Childs, D. S., O'Fallon, J. R. *et al.* (1969). Randomised controlled trial of adjuvant chemo-radiotherapy in completely resected gastric cancer. *The Lancet* **2**, 865–869.

Neri, B., Cini, G., Andreoli, F. *et al.* (2001). Randomised trial of adjuvant chemotherapy versus control after curative resection for gastric cancer: 5 year follow up. *British Journal of Cancer* **84**, 878–880.

Okajama K & Isozaki H. (1995). Splenectomy for treatment of gastric cancer: Japanese experience. *World Journal of Surgery* **19**, 537–540.

Parikh, D., Johnson, M., Chagia, L. *et al.* (1996). D2 gastrectomy: lessons from a prospective audit of the learning curve. *British Journal of Surgery* **83**, 1595–1599.

Seto, Y., Nagawa, H. & Muto, T. (1997). Results of extended lymph node dissection for gastric cancer cases with N2 lymph node metastases. *International Journal of Surgery* **82**, 257–261.

Siewert, J. R., Bottcher, K., Roder, J. D. *et al.* (1993). Prognostic relevance of systematic lymph node dissection in gastric carcinoma. *British Journal of Surgery* **80**, 1015–1018.

Siewert, J. R., Kestlemeier, R. & Busch, R. (1996). Benefits of gastric cancer and pNO pN1 lymph node metastases. *British Journal of Surgery* **83**, 1144–1147.

Smalley, S. R., Gunderson, L., Tepper, J. *et al.* (2001). Gastric surgical adjuvant radiotherapy consensus report: rationale and treatment implementation. *International Journal of Radiation Oncology, Biology, Physics* **52**, 283–293.

Sue-Ling, H. M., Johnson, D., Martin, I. G. *et al.* (1993). Gastric cancer: a curable disease in Britain. *British Medical Journal* **307**, 591–596.

Uno, Y., Obara, K., Kanazawa, K. *et al.* (1997). Stent implantation for malignant pyloric stenosis. *Gastrointestinal Endoscopy* **46**, 552–555.

Wanebo, H., Kennedy, B. J., Chmiel, J. *et al.* (1993). Cancer of the stomach: a patient care study by the American College of Surgeons. *Annals of Surgery* **218**, 583–592.

Wanebo, H. J., Kennedy, B. J., Winchester, D. P. *et al.* (1997). Role of splenectomy in gastric cancer surgery: an adverse effect of elective splenectomy on long-term survival. *Journal of American College of Surgeons* **185**, 177–184.

Zhang, Z. X. *et al.* (1998) Randomised clinical trial on the combination of pre-operative irradiation and surgery in the treatment of adenocarcinoma of gastric cardia- report on 370 patients. *International Journal of Radiation Oncology, Biology, Physics* **42**, 929–934.

Chapter 8

New targets in oesophago-gastric cancer

Nicholas C. Turner and Daniel Hochhauser

Introduction

Despite advances in diagnostic techniques, surgical management, radiotherapy and drug treatment of patients with oesophago-gastric (OG) cancer, most patients die of local recurrence or metastatic disease. It is therefore critically important to develop new strategies for the treatment of these cancers. Although radiotherapy and chemotherapy have a vital role in management, inherent and acquired resistance is a major problem. Increasing understanding of the molecular abnormalities that underlie the malignant process has led to the development of a host of rationally designed therapies. Many of these novel therapies may be relevant to OG tumours, and we review here some of the therapies being developed.

Circumvention of drug resistance

Although OG cancers may be initially sensitive to chemotherapy, the majority will become resistant to chemotherapy during treatment. Many mechanisms of drug resistance have been described and a detailed discussion is beyond the scope of this chapter. As described by Lowe, chemotherapy resistance can be thought of in terms of 'classical drug resistance' and 'down stream drug resistance' (Johnstone *et al.* 2002). We discuss some of the potential targets to circumvent drug resistance arising from these concepts.

Classical drug resistance

Classical drug resistance includes modulators of the drug–target interaction in cancer cells, and by interfering with this interaction inhibits the generation of damage within the cancer cell. There are several examples of classical drug resistance in OG cancer.

The efflux pumps form a family of drug resistance proteins that decrease the intracellular concentration of drug. Examples include P glycoprotein (PGP), and the multidrug resistance protein 1. Many different chemotherapy drugs can act as substrates for PGP, including the vinca-alkaloids and etoposide but not alkylating agents, and expression of PGP by the cell can lead to resistance to multiple drugs. Although the expression of PGP *in vitro* correlates with resistance of gastric cancer cell lines to chemotherapy (Endo *et al.* 1996), this has not been confirmed in clinical studies. Expression of PGP and multidrug resistance associated protein 1 had no impact on survival after adjuvant chemotherapy for gastric cancer (Choi *et al.* 2002).

A recent finding may explain this discrepancy in part. Other solid tumours, including those with low or absent 'resting' expression of PGP, will rapidly up-regulate the expression of PGP when exposed to chemotherapy (Abolhoda *et al.* 1999). Clinical studies may therefore underestimate the importance of PGP expression in solid tumours such as OG cancers. Several agents, such as the cyclosporin analogue PSC-833, are in development to interfere with the action of PGP and associated proteins aiming to enhance the efficacy of chemotherapy. There is some evidence of the efficacy of PSC-833 in treatment of acute myeloid leukaemia (Advani *et al.* 1999), but these agents have not yet been assessed in OG cancers. Many normal cells, such as bone-marrow stem cells and cells of the blood–brain barrier, express efflux pumps to protect against naturally occurring toxins presenting obvious difficulties to drug development.

Another important aspect of classical drug resistance is interference with the interaction of drug and target. Examples include alterations in folate transport and metabolism to circumvent the action of drugs such as 5-fluorouracil (5-FU), and methotrexate that inhibits DHFR. It has been reported that gastric cancers with high levels of the enzyme thymidylate synthetase (TS), the principal intra-cellular target of 5-FU, are resistant to 5-FU chemotherapy compared with cells expressing low levels of TS (Yeh *et al.* 1998). In contrast OG cancers expressing low levels of the topoisomerase II enzymes may be resistant to drugs that target topoisomerase II such as doxorubicin and etoposide which are used in the treatment of OG cancer (Rees *et al.* 2001). Repair of DNA damage may be important in chemotherapy resistance, for example DNA repair and resistance to cisplatin (Reed 1998), although the relative importance of DNA repair in chemotherapy resistance of OG cancers has not been established.

Downstream drug resistance

The cellular response to chemotherapy-induced DNA damage is a critical determinant of resistance to chemotherapy. Most chemotherapy drugs used in the treatment of OG cancers, either directly or indirectly, target DNA. The subsequent DNA damage is recognised by the cell, followed by selection of the appropriate response (Johnstone *et al.* 2002). These responses include decision to arrest the cell cycle to allow repair of DNA damage, or cell death by apoptosis. If the machinery in the cell responsible for detection of DNA damage, for the initiation of apoptosis, or for the orderly execution of apoptosis is defective then the cell may be resistant to chemotherapy.

There have been many mutations described in OG cancer that modulate these downstream processes. For example mutations in p53 are common in oesophageal cancers (Hollstein *et al.* 1991). The loss of functional p53 may allow the cell to continue to proliferate despite DNA damage, and oesophageal tumours with mutations in p53 are less responsive to chemoradiation (Ribeiro *et al.* 1998). The bcl-2 anti-apoptotic protein is also expressed in OG cancers (Ohbu *et al.* 1997; Muller *et al.* 1998). The role of bcl-2 in OG cancers is complex, with the protein expressed most commonly in early stage disease with expression correlating favourably with survival (Ohbu *et al.* 1997; Muller *et al.* 1998). This could be important in the application of strategies to target bcl-2, for example with bcl-2 antisense oligonucleotides (Webb *et al.* 1997).

Novel approaches to DNA targeting

The systemic administration of conventional chemotherapy is limited by the relative lack of tumour specificity and the ensuing systemic toxicity, with the dose of chemotherapy administered to the patient usually constrained by normal tissue tolerance. If novel chemotherapy drugs could be targeted to the tumour or the DNA damage limited to tumour cells, chemotherapy could be both better tolerated and more effective.

Hypoxia-activated drugs

Differences in the environment of a tumour as opposed to normal tissue may provide a non-specific method of targeting tumours. When tumours grow beyond a critical size the centre of the tumour becomes relatively hypoxic, and drugs that are activated in hypoxic conditions will in theory selectively target the tumour (Denny 2000). Examples of drugs in development include tirapazamine and the anthraquinone N-oxide AQ4N. Tirapazamine, when reduced in hypoxic conditions, induces DNA damage that at least in part is through poisoning topoisomerase II (Peters & Brown 2002). AQ4N, once activated by reduction, is also a potent inhibitor of topoisomerase II and may synergise with radiation and chemotherapy with little extra toxicity in normal, well-oxygenated, tissue (Patterson & McKeown 2000). Hypoxia has been demonstrated in oesophageal cancers (Kookourakis *et al.* 2001). Currently, early-phase studies are underway with AQ4N in combination with radiation for oesophageal cancers. However, there is potential for all hypoxia-targeted drugs to be less effective in clinical trials than *in vitro* and in animal experiments. The same deficiencies in vascularity and blood supply that lead to tumours becoming hypoxic may also hamper delivery of drug to target.

Sequence-specific DNA targeting

Conventional chemotherapy drugs have only limited sequence specificity, and novel drugs are in development with a higher degree of sequence specificity in their binding to DNA (Thurston 1999). These include novel cytotoxic drugs such as pyrrolobenzo-diazepine dimers that bind in the minor groove of DNA with a degree of sequence selectivity (Gregson *et al.* 2001). There is less efficient repair of drugs that cross-link DNA in the minor groove and such drugs are highly potent, one such drug (SJG-136) being 440-fold more potent than melphalan. Another approach is to develop drugs that are capable of binding to specific sequences of DNA with high affinity and artificially regulating gene expression by binding to promoter regulatory regions. Examples include the hairpin polyamides (O'Hare *et al.* 2002). This could allow inhibition of transcription factors implicated in drug resistance or tumour progression. Further development is required, as at present the number of nucleotides that these novel molecules can bind to is insufficient to allow any degree of clinically useful sequence selectivity.

Antibody-targeting strategies

Antibodies give a tumour-selective approach provided an epitope specific to tumour cells can be identified. Tumour-directed antibodies could either be used alone or as a delivery system. The use of antibodies to deliver toxins, drugs, radionucleotides, pro-drug activating enzymes or gene therapy has major theoretical benefits, although countless difficulties have been encountered in practice. An example of antibody-directed enzyme pro-drug therapy (ADEPT) uses a humanised monoclonal antibody specific for carcinoembryonic antigen (CEA) linked to an enzyme (Napier *et al.* 2000). After injection of the antibody–enzyme complex, the inert pro-drug is administered and is converted to active drug at the site of CEA-expressing tumours. CEA is expressed widely in OG cancers and clinical trials are underway.

Molecular targets

Current models of the perturbations cells undergo during malignant transformation have been well described by Hanahan & Weinberg (2000). Interference with one or more of these mutations may induce tumour stability or regression. An example of the potential efficacy of such a targeted approach comes from the use of imatinib (Kantarjian *et al.* 2002), a specific small molecule inhibitor of the tyrosine kinase *bcr-abl*, in chronic myeloid leukaemia (CML). By targeting the critical *bcr-abl* fusion protein in CML, imatinib is highly effective (O'Brien *et al.* 2003). There has been no single critical mutation identified in either gastric or oesophageal cancer, and the application of molecular targeted therapy may be a considerably more complex task in OG tumours. It is likely that combinations of chemotherapy and targeted therapies may be required to inhibit growth or induce apoptosis. Of the many potential targets, we discuss the targets that are closest to clinical trials.

Signal transduction

The most attractive pathways to target in the cell are the pathways typifying Hanahan and Weinberg's 'self-sufficiency in growth signals'. Cells are dependent on external growth factors to grow and suppress apoptosis. Cancer cells are characterised by deregulation of growth factor pathways overriding normal cellular dependence on extracellular growth factors, and enhancing cellular proliferation. The growth factor receptor with the greatest relevance to OG cancer is the epidermal growth factor receptor (EGFR). EGFR is a receptor tyrosine kinase that is over-expressed in squamous oesophageal tumours (Lu *et al.* 1988) and in up to 80% of gastric cancers (Slesak *et al.* 1998). EGFR links to downstream signal transduction pathways such as the *ras–raf–mapk* kinase signal transduction pathway, although to view this as a single linear pathway is a simplification as cross-talk between alternative pathways occurs at nearly every level. The ultimate effects of the activation of this pathway are also multiple. Although it is clear that the pathway is capable of inducing cell proliferation by altering the expression of the cyclins, cyclin-dependent kinases (CDK) and cyclin-dependent kinase inhibitors (CDKI), the pathway also modulates apoptosis and angiogenesis.

Growth factor receptors

There are several approaches to blocking the EGFR in OG tumours. One approach uses antibodies, such as cetuximab (Erbitux) (C-225), that bind to the extracellular domain of EGFR and inhibit the activation of the receptor. Alternative approaches use small molecules, such as gefitinib (Iressa) (ZD1839) and erlotinib (Tarceva) (OSI-774), to target the tyrosine kinase on the intracellular domain. These agents prevent dimerisation of the receptor and this prevents activation of the downstream effectors. There are encouraging data from animal models that targeting EGFR may be an effective strategy in gastric cancer, with a blocking monoclonal antibody to the EGFR inhibiting the growth of human gastric cancer xenografts in nude mice (Teramoto *et al.* 1996).

Although there are few clinical data on the use of the small molecule EGFR tyrosine kinase inhibitors in OG cancer, there are encouraging data on the use of gefitinib (ZD-1839) in non-small-cell lung cancer (NSCLC) with disease responses as a single agent (Herbst *et al.* 2002). Despite the observed synergy of ZD-1839 with platinum chemotherapy *in vitro* (Ciardiello *et al.* 2000), there was no demonstrable advantage in the addition of ZD-1839 to first-line chemotherapy for NSCLC *in vivo* (ESMO 2002). This underlies the importance of understanding the mechanisms of synergy between receptor tyrosine kinase inhibitors and chemotherapy. Antagonism of the EGFR in oesophageal cancer cells *in vitro* enhances chemotherapy-induced apoptosis (Nguyen *et al.* 2002), but it remains to be seen how effective such strategies will be in the clinic. At present, there are no known biochemical or molecular predictors of response to these agents, which only reinforces the current lack of understanding of their mode of action.

Ras–raf–MAP kinase

There have been several different approaches developed to interfere with the function of the *ras–raf–MAP* kinase pathway. These approaches have recently been reviewed by Downward (2003). Interestingly, mutations in the *ras* genes are surprisingly uncommon in the OG cancers (Hollstein *et al.* 1991), and it remains unclear how valuable inhibition of this pathway will be in OG cancer.

Cyclins and CDKs

Mutations in the genes involved in the G1/S phase transition are common in OG cancers. For example in oesophageal cancer common events include downregulation of Rb (Jiang *et al.* 1993), cyclin D1 amplification (Jiang *et al.* 1993) and silencing of the cyclin dependent kinase inhibitor p16 by promoter hypermethylation (Xing *et al.* 1999).

Drugs that inhibit the CDKs may arrest the cell cycle and inhibit tumour growth. Although CDK inhibitors such as flavopiridol have activity *in vitro* on oesophageal adenocarcinoma cell lines (Schrump *et al.* 1998), there was no evidence of significant activity in a phase II study of patients with advanced gastric adenocarcinomas (Schwartz *et al.* 2001).

An alternative approach to blocking CDKs is to enhance the action of endogenous CDKIs. An example such an approach, which at least in part acts by increasing CDKI levels, are the proteasome inhibitors. CDKIs are degraded in the cell by the proteasomes after ubiquitination of CDKIs by the ubiquitination enzymes. Inhibitors of proteasome function, such as PS-341 and MG132, may induce cell cycle arrest by elevating CDKI levels. Proteasome inhibitors will have a wider range of effects on cellular proteins than solely by elevating cellular concentration of the CDKIs, and there is also evidence to support an effect on p53 and pro-apoptotic proteins. Proteasome inhibitors have demonstrated some evidence of activity in gastric cancer cell lines *in vitro* (Fan *et al.* 2001), although there are as yet no clinical data.

Cyclooxygenase II inhibitors

Cyclooxygenase II (COX 2) is commonly expressed in oesophageal squamous tumours, and selective COX-2 inhibitors suppress proliferation and enhancing apoptosis in these cells *in vitro* (Zimmermann *et al.* 1999). Reinforced by recent evidence that long-term aspirin can reduce the incidence of colonic polyps (Sandler *et al.* 2003), the inhibition of COX-2 remains a potential target in the OG cancers.

Assumptions of novel therapies

There are assumptions for novel targeted therapies that in practice may prove to be incorrect. These include:

- *Resistance is less likely to develop.* The use chemotherapy in OG cancers is limited by resistance, either inherent or acquired, but it has been assumed that resistance to targeted therapies would be hard to acquire. Recent evidence from the use of imatinib in CML suggests otherwise, and resistance to imatinib can develop secondary to mutations in the *abl* kinase (Gorre *et al.* 2001). With greater use of targeted therapies it is likely that further examples will arise.
- *Targeting will reduce toxicity.* A therapeutic window clearly exists in the use of drugs such as imatinib and gefitinib with relatively little toxicity. However, to view

targeted therapies as free of side effects would be incorrect with the potential for unexpected toxicity, as for example in reports of gefitinib-induced interstitial pneumonia (Inoue *et al.* 2003).

• *The situation in vitro will correspond with the situation in vivo.* The effectiveness of novel therapies *in vitro* may not translate to effectiveness *in vivo*. Perhaps the best example of this is the synergy of iressa and chemotherapy *in vitro*, and the lack of synergy demonstrated *in vivo*.

Conclusion

Novel therapies in development hold great promise for the treatment of OG cancers. We are some way from understanding how to apply these therapies in practice, and a greater understanding of the complexities of molecular pathways is required. Rather than tackle the tumour with a single, novel therapy, it is likely that the best results will come from combinations of novel therapies, possibly alongside conventional therapies. How the optimum combination will be selected on a tumour-by-tumour basis is currently not clear, although the answer is likely to come with advances in genomics and proteomics.

References

Abolhoda, A., Wilson, A. E., Ross, H. *et al.* (1999). Rapid activation of MDR1 gene expression in human metastatic sarcoma after in vivo exposure to doxorubicin. *Clinical Cancer Research* **5**, 3352–3356.

Advani, R., Saba, H. I., Tallman, M. S. *et al.* (1999). Treatment of refractory and relapsed acute myelogenous leukemia with combination chemotherapy plus the multidrug resistance modulator PSC 833 (Valspodar). *Blood* **93**, 787–795.

Chene, P. (2003). Inhibiting the p53-MDM2 interaction: an important target for cancer therapy. *Nature Reviews Cancer* **3**, 102–109.

Choi, J. H., Lim, H. Y., Joo, H. J. *et al.* (2002). Expression of multidrug resistance-associated protein1, P-glycoprotein, and thymidylate synthase in gastric cancer patients treated with 5-fluorouracil and doxorubicin-based adjuvant chemotherapy after curative resection. *British Journal of Cancer* **86**, 1578–1585.

Ciardiello, F., Caputo, R., Bianco, R. *et al.* (2000). Antitumor effect and potentiation of cytotoxic drugs activity in human cancer cells by ZD-1839 (Iressa), an epidermal growth factor receptor-selective tyrosine kinase inhibitor. *Clinical Cancer Research* **6**, 2053–2063.

Denny, W. A. (2000). The role of hypoxia-activated prodrugs in cancer therapy. *The Lancet Oncology* **1**, 25–29.

Downward, J. (2003). Targeting RAS signalling pathways in cancer therapy. *Nature Reviews Cancer* **3**, 11–22.

Endo, K., Maehara, Y., Kusumoto, T. *et al.* (1996). Expression of multidrug-resistance-associated protein (MRP) and chemosensitivity in human gastric cancer. *International Journal of Cancer* **68**, 372–377.

Fan, X. M., Wong, B. C., Wang, W. P. *et al.* (2001). Inhibition of proteasome function induced apoptosis in gastric cancer. *International Journal of Cancer* **93**, 481–488.

Gorre, M. E., Mohammed, M., Ellwood, K. *et al.* (2001). Clinical resistance to STI-571 cancer therapy caused by BCR-ABL gene mutation or amplification. *Science* **293**, 876–880.

Gregson, S. J., Howard, P. W., Hartley, J. A. *et al.* (2001). Design, synthesis, and evaluation of a novel pyrrolobenzodiazepine DNA-interactive agent with highly efficient cross-linking ability and potent cytotoxicity. *Journal of Medical Chemistry* **44**, 737–748.

Hanahan, D. & Weinberg, R. A. (2000). The hallmarks of cancer. *Cell* **100**, 57–70.

Herbst, R. S., Maddox, A. M., Rothenberg, M. L. *et al.* (2002). Selective oral epidermal growth factor receptor tyrosine kinase inhibitor ZD1839 is generally well-tolerated and has activity in non-small-cell lung cancer and other solid tumors: results of a phase I trial. *Journal of Clinical Oncology* **20**, 3815–3825.

Hollstein, M. C., Peri, L., Mandard, A. M., Welsh, J. A., Montesano, R., Metcalf, R. A., Bak, M. & Harris, C. C. (1991). Genetic analysis of human esophageal tumors from two high incidence geographic areas: frequent p53 base substitutions and absence of ras mutations. *Cancer Research* **51**, 4102–4106.

Inoue, A., Saijo, Y., Maemondo, M., Gomi, K., Tokue, Y., Kimura, Y., Ebina, M., Kikuchi, T., Moriya, T. & Nukiwa, T. (2003). Severe acute interstitial pneumonia and gefitinib. *The Lancet* **361**, 137–139.

Jiang, W., Zhang, Y. J., Kahn, S. M. *et al.* (1993). Altered expression of the cyclin D1 and retinoblastoma genes in human esophageal cancer. *Proceedings of the National Academy of Sciences of the United States of America* **90**, 9026–9030.

Johnstone, R. W., Ruefli, A. A. & Lowe, S. W. (2002). Apoptosis: a link between cancer genetics and chemotherapy. *Cell* **108**, 153–164.

Kantarjian, H., Sawyers, C., Hochhaus, A *et al.* (2002). Hematologic and cytogenetic responses to imatinib mesylate in chronic myelogenous leukemia. *New England Journal of Medicine* **346**, 645–652.

Koukourakis, M.I., Giatromanolaki, A., Skarlatos, J. *et al.* (2001). Hypoxia inducible factor (HIF-1a and HIF-2a) expression in early esophageal cancer and response to photodynamic therapy and radiotherapy. *Cancer Research* **61**, 1830–1832.

Lu, S. H., Hsieh, L. L., Luo, F.C. & Weinstein, I. B. (1988). Amplification of the EGF receptor and c-myc genes in human esophageal cancers. *International Journal of Cancer* **42**, 502–505.

Muller, W., Schneiders, A., Hommel, G. & Gabbert, H. E. (1998). Prognostic value of bcl-2 expression in gastric cancer. *Anticancer Research* **18**(6B), 4699–4704.

Napier, M. P., Sharma, S. K., Springer, C. J., Bagshawe, K. D., Green, A. J., Martin, J., Stribbling, S. M., Cushen, N., O'Malley, D. & Begent, R. H. (2000). Antibody-directed enzyme prodrug therapy: efficacy and mechanism of action in colorectal carcinoma. *Clinical Cancer Research* **6**, 765–772.

Nguyen, D. M., Chen, A. & Stewart, J. H. *et al.* (2002). The erbB1 antagonist PD153035 (PD) inhibits DNA repair and potentiates cisplatin- or radiation-induced apoptosis in esophageal cancer (EsC) cells. *Proceedings of the American Association for Cancer Research*, **43**, abstract 4970.

O'Brien, S. G., Guilhot, F., Larson, R. A. *et al.* (2003). Imatinib compared with interferon and low-dose cytarabine for newly diagnosed chronic-phase chronic myeloid leukemia. *New England Journal of Medicine* **348**, 994–1004.

O'Hare, C.C., Mack, D., Tandon, M. *et al.* (2002). DNA sequence recognition in the minor groove by crosslinked polyamides: The effect of N-terminal head group and linker length on binding affinity and specificity. *Proceedings of the National Academy of Sciences of the United States of America* **99**, 72–77.

Ohbu, M., Saegusa, M., Kobayashi, N. *et al.* (1997). Expression of bcl-2 protein in esophageal squamous cell carcinomas and its association with lymph node metastasis. *Cancer* **79**, 1287–1293.

Patterson, L. H. & McKeown, S. R. (2000). AQ4N: a new approach to hypoxia-activated cancer chemotherapy. *British Journal of Cancer* **83**, 1589–1593.

Peters, K. B. & Brown, J. M. (2002). Tirapazamine: a hypoxia-activated topoisomerase II poison. *Cancer Research* **62**, 5248–5253.

Reed, E. (1998). Platinum-DNA adduct, nucleotide excision repair and platinum based anti-cancer chemotherapy. *Cancer Treatment Reviews* **24**, 331–344.

Rees, M., Stahl, M., Klump, B., Willers, R., Gabbert, H. E. & Sarbia, M. (2001). The prognostic significance of proliferative activity, apoptosis and expression of DNA topoisomerase II alpha in multimodally-treated oesophageal squamous cell carcinoma. *Anticancer Research* **21**, 3637–3642.

Ribeiro, U. Jr, Finkelstein, S. D., Safatle-Ribeiro, A. V. *et al.* (1998). p53 sequence analysis predicts treatment response and outcome of patients with esophageal carcinoma. *Cancer* **83**, 7–18.

Sandler, R. S., Halabi, S., Baron, J. A. *et al.* (2003). A randomized trial of aspirin to prevent colorectal adenomas in patients with previous colorectal cancer. *New England Journal of Medicine* **348**, 883–890.

Schrump, D. S., Matthews, W., Chen, G. A., Mixon, A. & Altorki, N. K. (1998). Flavopiridol mediates cell cycle arrest and apoptosis in esophageal cancer cells. *Clinical Cancer Research* **4**, 2885–2890.

Schwartz, G. K., Ilson, D., Saltz, L. *et al.* (2001). Phase II study of the cyclin-dependent kinase inhibitor flavopiridol administered to patients with advanced gastric carcinoma. *Journal of Clinical Oncology* **19**, 1985–1992.

Slesak, B., Harlozinska, A., Porebska, I. *et al.* (1998). Expression of epidermal growth factor receptor family proteins (EGFR, c-erbB-2 and c-erbB-3) in gastric cancer and chronic gastritis. *Anticancer Research* **18**(4A), 2727–2732.

Teramoto, T., Onda, M., Tokunaga, A. & Asano, G. (1996). Inhibitory effect of anti-epidermal growth factor receptor antibody on a human gastric cancer. *Cancer* **77**(8 Suppl.), 1639–1645.

Thurston, D. E. (1999). Nucleic acid targeting: therapeutic strategies for the 21st century. *British Journal of Cancer* **80** (Suppl. 1), 65–85.

van Oosterom, A. T., Judson, I., Verweij, J. *et al.* (2001). Safety and efficacy of imatinib (STI571) in metastatic gastrointestinal stromal tumours: a phase I study. *The Lancet* **358**, 1421–1423.

Webb, A., Cunningham, D., Cotter, F. *et al.* (1997). BCL-2 antisense therapy in patients with non-Hodgkin lymphoma. *The Lancet* **349**, 1137–1141.

Xing, E. P., Nie, Y., Wang, L. D., Yang, G. Y. & Yang, C. S. (1999). Aberrant methylation of p16INK4a and deletion of p15INK4b are frequent events in human esophageal cancer in Linxian, China. *Carcinogenesis* **20**, 77–84.

Yeh, K. H., Shun, C. T., Chen, C. L. *et al.* (1998). High expression of thymidylate synthase is associated with the drug resistance of gastric carcinoma to high dose 5-fluorouracil-based systemic chemotherapy. *Cancer* **82**, 1626–1631.

Zimmermann, K. C., Sarbia, M., Weber, A. A. *et al.* (1999). Cyclooxygenase-2 expression in human esophageal carcinoma. *Cancer Research* **59**, 198–204.

PART 3

Pancreatic cancer and cancer of the biliary tract

Pancreatic head tumours: diagnosis and assessment for surgery with curative intent

Satvinder S. Mudan

Introduction

Pancreatic cancer remains one of the most formidable of challenges in surgical oncology. As other chapters in this volume demonstrate, the management of pancreatic cancer challenges, to the fullest, skills of the diagnostician, surgical oncologist, medical oncologist and the palliative care workers; it remains the Everest of solid tumours (DiMagno *et al.* 1999).

Diagnosis in pancreatic cancer presents its own specific problems and we shall discuss these before dealing with the selection of patients to undergo radical surgical intervention. In doing so, we introduce a notion of selection for operation with curative intent. By this term, we presuppose that there exists a potential to cure pancreatic cancer surgically or at the very least alter the tumour behaviour, and moreover that such a cure relies on the complete ablation of loco-regional disease through achieving R0 resection, which is the absence of untreated residual disease and completely clear margins in the resection specimen. Patients undergoing less than R0 resection, i.e. those patients with positive resection margins (R1) or those with macroscopic residual disease (R2) fare no better that those receiving palliative therapies alone. Previously, assessment for resection in pancreatic cancer was a technical feasibility exercise rather than an attempt to conclude whether an oncologically effective resection might be possible.

Technical limitations to surgery such as involvement of the portal venous system or the regional arteries have been overcome but do not necessarily translate into an oncologic benefit to the patient. We know that recurrence after 'successful' surgery is common and that the tumour-specific mortality of pancreatic cancer is nearly unity. It would seem undeniably obvious that surgery alone is insufficient as treatment but may form the platform for systemic therapies. The patterns of failure suggest that the selection of patients for surgery misses a substantial number of patients with 'occult' distant or peritoneal disease and surgical pathology data demonstrate that positive margins are commonplace, even in the best centres.

The nature of the operations is complex and even in the best centres it is not uncommon that an unexpected intra-operative finding at laparotomy will preclude the operation proceeding. This is demoralising for the patient who still has to recover from a painful upper abdominal incision and may yet yield to surgical complications.

Complication rates for resectional surgery are high compared with other operations and although mortality rates have fallen considerably over the years this is a function of improved postoperative care and salvage rather than a decline in the surgical complication rates (Kotwall *et al.* 2002).

It is thought that by increasing the volume-per-centre improvement in operative and oncologic outcome can be achieved. The former is a construct based on infrastructure and medical skill base and has some evidence to support it. However, the latter premise can only be assumed if the ability to select patients for intervention is also enhanced.

If only a few patients are suitable for operation and, even amongst these, cures are not commonplace how do we best select and focus our resources on these few and as a corollary reduce effort on those where surgery is unlikely to be helpful and better divert the patient to appropriate palliative therapies? Indeed, surgery which is undertaken but cannot be completed or results in positive margins, may have a detrimental effect on the patient's physical status and thus prognosis. Time to death from diagnosis in inoperable pancreatic cancer is in the range of 6 months and the not infrequent complications of surgery and even the morbidity of just a laparotomy wound may keep the patient in hospital for many weeks denying the patient valuable time with his family. Consequently, palliation is the correct treatment pathway for most (~90%) patients, and careful patient selection for potentially curative surgical intervention is critical.

In this chapter we will discuss the management of pancreatic cancer from diagnosis to selection for operation and in particular the criteria for inoperability that present hurdles to successful operation and the methods by which we can hope to identify these criteria in the patient.

In taking a patient from a diagnostic scan to operation it is necessary to be confident as possible that the patient will benefit from operation. Appropriate discussions can take place regarding risk and benefit, patients unlikely to benefit can be spared an unnecessary laparotomy and resources deployed most effectively. How such a strategy is affected by one's approach to palliation is also discussed.

Diagnosis

Clinical presentation

Clinical suspicion should be aroused in a patient greater than 40 years of age who presents, especially if a heavy smoker, with any of the following: obstructive jaundice, unexplained weight loss of greater than 10%, unexplained lumbar or epigastric pain, unexplained dyspepsia, a non-obese patient with sudden onset of diabetes in the absence of a family history, steatorrhoea, several attacks of idiopathic pancreatitis. Although not conclusive, certain occupational groups such as chemical and petrochemical, dye and rubber industry workers are thought to be at greater risk. Pancreatic cancer in a first-degree relative increases the relative risk (RR) by 13 and there are associations with hereditary cancer syndromes such as familial adenomatous polyposis (FAP) syndrome (RR 4.46) and familial atypical multiple mole melanoma FAMMM syndrome with p16 abnormality (RR 13) (Everhart and Wright 1995; Gold and Goldin 1998; Dimagno *et al.* 1999).

Most (>80%) cases of periampullary cancer present with jaundice but other symptoms are usually concurrent. The classical description of jaundice without any pain is not common and careful enquiry reveals that epigastric pain is frequent (>75%) but is of a constant and boring quality in contradistinction to biliary colic and weight loss is the rule (>85%) (Janes *et al.* 1996). Backache is not infrequent but is more commonly a feature of cancers in the body of pancreas rather than the head and often indicates inoperability due to locally advanced disease. Steatorrhoea and painless jaundice are associated with resectability and better outcome.

In advanced disease cachexia and ascites may be present. Paraneoplastic phenomena such as intestinal dysmotility manifesting as gastroparesis and prolonged intestinal transit times may be present (Barkin *et al.* 1986). Hypercoagulability may present as thrombophlebitis migrans and autopsy series report an incidence of about 17% of deep venous thrombosis (Rickles & Edwards 1983).

Diagnostic tools

Endoscopic retrograde cholangiopancreatography (ERCP) can be used as a diagnostic modality as the appearance of a pancreatic cancer is often classical at ERCP. A 'double duct' sign showing occlusion of both the pancreatic duct and distal bile duct on the head of pancreas is considered as diagnostic of pancreatic head cancer. Parenchymal abnormality can only be inferred and a normal pancreatogram does not exclude malignancy (Hewitt *et al.* 1998). Moreover, the technique has 'silent areas' for the uncinate and small ampullary lesions. The role of ERCP in the diagnosis of pancreatic cancer has diminished to the point that it is no longer indicated in the diagnostic sequence. As a therapeutic tool in the management of pancreatic head cancer, ERCP has an important role in the relief of jaundice for the inoperable patient. It is of less value in pancreatic body tumours which typically do not present with jaundice. In a patient considered inoperable because of obvious distant disease or medically unfit then ERCP can be therapeutic by placement of endobiliary stent to relieve jaundice. Placement of a stent interferes with staging by causing additional inflammation in the hepatic ligament and local lymphadenopathy. Most surgeons would prefer not only that staging is complete before consideration of stenting but to operate without stent placement (Povoski *et al.* 1999). However, for a variety of pragmatic reasons, it may not be possible to complete the staging sequence speedily and so stenting with a plastic stent to relieve the jaundice may be preferable to leaving the patient in a jaundiced condition. A metallic stent should not be placed until and if the patient is definitely not to be considered for surgical resection.

At present, diagnosis relies on the relevant history in conjunction with imaging modalities of trans-cutaneous ultrasound, computed tomography (CT) scan, magnetic resonance imaging (MRI), endoscopic ultrasound (EUS) and positron emission tomography (PET) scanning (Clarke *et al.* 2003). In early disease a mass may not be evident on imaging and even if a mass is seen in the periampullary region one cannot immediately determine whether the tumour is benign or malignant, the clinical history may guide the careful enquirer. Careful ultrasound can be very sensitive but confounders such as body habitus, overlying bowel gas and user dependence result in inadequate examinations in 20–30% of cases (Trede *et al.* 1997). Dual-phase spiral CT scan produces reliability and reproducibility across institutions and users. The ubiquity of CT scan, rapid image acquisition and processing times make CT an indispensable tool and in general first choice investigation for pancreatic diagnosis. The sensitivity and specificity are high (>95%) for tumours 3 cm or greater in dimension but diminish to about 70% for tumours less than 2 cm (Schwarz *et al.* 2001). MRI has advantages of non-ionizing radiation but MRI experience is less common, acquisition and processing times are considerably longer and small masses are less detectable. Where a lesion is demonstrated but its nature presents a problem MR may have superiority over CT in this qualitative discussion and usually this will apply only to small potentially inflammatory masses or rare neoplastic lesions of the pancreas such as intraductal papillary mucinous tumors (IPMTs) (Sahani *et al.* 2002).

EUS yields superb sensitivity for pancreatic masses and anatomic detail and is the modality of choice for small or suspected tumours. Several studies show the superiority of EUS over CT in lesions under 2 cm in size (Legmann *et al.* 1998; Midwinter *et al.* 1999; Schwarz *et al.* 2001). The specificity of EUS is less than that of CT and the sensitivity of CT for smaller lesions is improving. The future role of EUS is more likely to be in targeted tissue biopsy where this is felt indicated (see later).

PET scanning is still developing and, although the sensitivity is not better than CT, MRI or EUS, specificity is superior. A study from Duke University Medical Center, Durham, North Carolina, found specificity for pancreatic cancer of 86% and 62% for PET and CT scan, respectively (Kaladay *et al.* 2002).

The tumour marker CA19.9 may be elevated and a threshold value of 200 U/ml yields 95% specificity. Caution should be exercised in the presence of deep jaundice where impaired degradation of CA19.9 in the liver leads to false positive results and in Lewis blood groups a or b where false negatives can occur. However, the combination of convincing history, raised CA19.9 and CT detected mass has a specificity of close to 100% (Mann *et al.* 2000). Failure to normalise the CA19.9 after relief of jaundice should be considered with great suspicion for cancer.

Two single-institution studies of multimodal evaluation of potential pancreatic cancer patients, from hospitals with a major interest in pancreatic cancer, support the use of CT scan as the primary diagnostic tool (Schwarz *et al.* 2001; Del Frate 2002).

Whether a malignant mass arises from the pancreas, the distal bile duct or ampulla of Vater can be difficult to establish. The pathological site may become apparent after resection and close pathologic examination of the specimen. Prognosis varies with the exact site and so has important implications but may be impossible to determine even in the resected specimen. Highly sensitive examinations such as EUS may help clarify this question, but often may not. Initial work up and treatment planning are not different and so one can consider the clinical problem to be of a periampullary tumour rather than a specific site.

Role of biopsy

The diagnosis of pancreatic cancer based on clinical history, physical findings, CT scan and CA19.9 has a predictive value of about 95–98%. This means that there is a false-positive rate of about 5%. CT or ultrasound-guided needle biopsy can be used for confirmation of the diagnosis. However, there are several theoretical and some practical limitations to needle biopsy. There is a theoretical possibility of cancer-cell dissemination into the peritoneal cavity but the evidence that this has any impact on the natural history of the disease is very scant. There are anecdotal examples of needle tract seeding but again whether this has a significant effect on the natural history is questionable. In both cases these theoretical disadvantages of diagnostic biopsy could be mitigated by transduodenal biopsy under EUS guidance. The major argument against percutaneous or transduodenal biopsy is the poor sensitivity of the biopsy. Pancreatic cancers can be small and yet induce a great deal of peritumoral fibrosis. Thus biopsy is technically difficult and false negative biopsy is not uncommon. Serial biopsy in suspected cancer delays treatment and may do so to a point that operation with curative intent is no longer possible but the diagnosis more obvious. Most pancreatic centres do not advocate preoperative biopsy in potentially operable candidates except where there is substantial clinical doubt in the diagnosis. Only once the patient has been deemed inoperable should biopsy normally be considered.

If ERCP is to be undertaken then bile may be sampled at the ERCP or brush cytology taken. If cancer cells are seen in the bile this confirms the diagnosis of a periampullary cancer. Usually it is not possible to determine whether the cancer cells have originated from a distal bile duct cancer or the pancreatic duct. As ever, a negative test cannot imply the reverse.

Assessment for operation

Several components merge in the assessment of a patient for resection of a pancreatic cancer. The operations are large and demanding on the patient's baseline medical condition. The demographics of the disease dictate that many of the patients will be elderly and fragile. In general, age and tumour size are not a contraindication to operation but extra-regional disease, tumour biology and co-morbidities might be (Fong *et al.* 1995; Huguier & Mason 1999). In this way we suggest that the notion of assessment for operation is different from staging of the tumour. Staging implies an anatomic description of the extent of disease but does not take into account the disease behaviour or tumour biology and no account of patient characteristics. Whereas staging and resectibility can be measured objectively, 'operability' has a more subjective overlay that implies a degree of surgical experience in addition to the use of recognised anaesthetic-risk assessment tools. Both are necessary for patient selection in pancreatic cancer surgery.

In the diagnostic phase of assessing the patient, imaging may well demonstrate features of inoperability such as rapidly progressive disease, cachexia and clinical ascites. Patients who present without jaundice are much less likely to be resectable than those who do (Kalser *et al.* 1985), similarly for pain (Kelsen *et al.*1997).

Resection of distant sites such as liver and resection of major vascular structures is all possible but has been shown not to carry benefit to the patient, thus the patient can be resectable but inoperable for features of the extent of disease that suggest a poor tumour biology. Accepted criteria of inoperability are as follows.

Absolute contraindications.
* Distant disease and in the pancreas this is most commonly the liver although 30–40% have pulmonary disease, 20% adrenal metastases and 6–9% ovarian metastases.
* Arterial involvement usually by encasement of the coeliac and its branches and or the superior mesenteric artery.
* Obvious peritoneal metastases.

Relative contraindications.
* Involvement of the mesenterico-porto-splenic venous system.
* Nodal disease has a significant adverse effect on prognosis and nodal disease at distant sites such as the coeliac axis and para-aortic region carries the same biological significance as distant metastatic disease.

Imaging to evaluate expeditiously these criteria of inoperability is crucial in the clinical pathway. The surgeon needs to identify patients with inoperability criteria as defined above so that they can be diverted to a palliative pathway. Within the palliative group the surgeon needs to stratify patients based on the likely survival characteristics and determine the most appropriate palliative therapy (Schwarz & Beger 2000). Patients with metastatic disease to the liver and or the parietes typically have survival times of 3–6 months (Fujino *et al.* 2003). This applies also to occult peritoneal disease in the form of positive peritoneal cytology. Positive peritoneal cytology is usually only seen in large tumours and almost without exception there are also other criteria of inoperability (Lei *et al.* 1994; Jimenez *et al.* 2000). Patients deemed inoperable owing to reasons of nodal disease outside of the resection field or vascular involvement beyond that which can be encompassed by a limited vein resection have longer survival times, approaching about one year. Approximately half of the patients deemed inoperable at laparotomy fall into the latter group and half into the former (Luque-de Leon *et al.* 1999; Barreiro *et al.* 2002). Combined, this inoperable group comprises about 20-30% of all, otherwise 'good-risk' patients coming to operation having been deemed resectable on CT criteria alone (Trede *et al.* 1997; Diehl 1998; McCarthy *et al.* 1998; Midwinter *et al.* 1999; Nieveen van Dijkum 2003). Therefore several sites require careful evaluation namely the liver, the peritoneal surfaces, nodal stations and the local vasculature. No single imaging modality in isolation yields a sufficiently accurate picture to establish operability.

Clinical presentation and medical fitness

Patients diagnosed with pancreatic cancer who do not present with jaundice are far less likely to be resectable. Pain and in particular back pain is said to be associated with irresectibility and poor outcome. Kelsen *et al.* (1997) found that pain was a significant predictor of survival outcome in both resected and irresectable patients. Prolonged jaundice and possibly even episodes of cholangitis mean the patients are not uncommonly nutritionally wasted at the time of assessment. Whether pre-operative nutritional support is of value in this group is as yet an unanswered question.

Extra-abdominal disease

The evaluation of metastatic sites from pancreatic cancer relates to the liver as the main site of visceral metastases. However, the incidence of pulmonary metastases is 30% and another 7% of patients will have mediastinal nodal metastases without evidence of visceral lung metastases. Other sites of metastatic disease such as adrenal and ovary are also common in autopsy series (Lee & Tatter 1984; Hahn & Faigel 2001). Improvements in extracorporeal imaging should identify most of these but in questionable cases where the primary seems to be advanced a case can be made for PET scan although most studies seem to show that the addition of PET scan while contributing to a more precise extent-of-disease evaluation does not lead to an alteration in the management strategy (Diedrichs *et al.* 2000; Kalady *et al.* 2002). If we perform EUS for pancreatic cancer, then we do search for mediastinal disease but currently do not routinely perform PET scans.

Vascular assessment

Although we would consider arterial infiltration to be an absolute contraindication to operation, venous involvement is a relative issue. Past studies of 'regional pancreatectomy' involving arterial resection and reconstruction showed high mortality without survival benefit (Sindelar 1989). Where portal vein resection is performed to achieve negative margins because of tumour adhesion to the vein, the survivorship in this group appears to match that where venous resection was not required to gain negative margins, and contrasts with those in whom there is transmural invasion of the vein where survivorship matches those with inoperable disease (Reber & Gloor 1998; Harrison & Brennan 1998; Jurowich *et al.* 2000; Shibata *et al.* 2001). Evolution in CT scan technology, from conventional CT through dual-phase spiral CT and to CT angiography with multidetector scanners, has improved the sensitivity for vascular involvement either of the vein or artery and is equivalent or even superior to MR-angiography, with good CT taking the sensitivity and specificity to about 90% and 100%, respectively. Both these modalities exceed the performance of either EUS or conventional percutaneous angiography (Diehl *et al.* 1998; Legmann *et al.* 1998; McCarthy *et al.* 1998; Novick & Fishman 1998; Midwinter *et al.* 1999; Horton 2002) and without the need of an invasive test. Consequently, percutaneous transcatheter angiography has been dropped in the paradigm of pancreatic cancer staging in most institutions and EUS is not thought to have sufficient sensitivity and specificity for clinical practice in assessment of venous invasion (Rosch *et al.* 2000).

More detailed study of the portal venous system is possible by intraportal ultrasonography and can aid in the separation of tumour adhesion and mural invasion. However, this is available in only a few centres and awaits evaluation as a part of the staging process (Kaneko *et al.* 1998).

Nodal disease

Enlarged inflammatory nodes are frequent in pancreatic cancer, especially if the patient has been stented. In a study comparing EUS, CT and MRI the sensitivity was 68, 59 and 77%, respectively (Cannon *et al.* 1999). However, the specificity for all these modalities tends to be higher (~90%) than the sensitivity (Midwinter *et al.* 1999). Patients with nodal disease in distant sites such as the para-aortic region tend to have a poor prognosis despite resection and histological proof of this may render an otherwise resectable patient inoperable. The sensitivity of PET scan for nodes close to the tumour is poor although more useful in evaluating distant nodes. Although the specificity is high it is not thought to be sufficiently high enough to alter the decision to operate based on PET findings alone. (Kalady *et al.* 2002; Valinas *et al.* 2002). Nodal staging is probably most precisely obtained by skilled EUS (Schwarz *et al.* 2001) and in addition has the potential that nodes lying outside the field of a conventional operation and which might declare the patient inoperable can be biopsied. EUS-guided needle-biopsy provides the best tool to meet this staging option. Both the sensitivity and specificity for this modality are high compared with extracorporeal imaging (Midwinter *et al.* 1999).

Assessment of the liver and peritoneal surfaces

The patterns of failure in pancreatic cancer suggest that about 60% of patients have liver metastases not detected by CT scan and 60% have occult peritoneal disease (Lee & Tatter 1984; Sperti *et al.* 1997; Luque-de Leon *et al.* 1999). Subcapsular, subcentimetre metastases are typical of periampullary cancers. Consequently, most recurrences after operation are intra-abdominal and in about one third of all patients, whether resected with curative intent or not, cancer related death will eventually be by a combination of serosal and liver disease. A further third will recur by liver disease alone and the remaining third by loco-regional disease.

Small-volume liver disease and small peritoneal deposits are a major source of non-therapeutic or 'open-and-close' laparotomy. In our experience local extension of tumour into the small bowel mesentery in the region of the ligament of Trietz is not an uncommon finding and is undetectable at CT even if symptoms of duodenal obstruction are present.

Despite the improvements in technology the major sources of failure to detect a cause of inoperability are small volume liver and peritoneal metastases that typify pancreatic cancer. The sensitivity of good CT or MRI for small-volume peritoneal/liver disease is about 70–80% (Diehl *et al.* 1998).

The value of PET scan suggests a sensitivity of about 60% at best and falls to 40% for peritoneal metastases below 1 cm diameter (Kalady *et al.* 2002). PET scan sensitivity for intrahepatic lesions is good for lesions greater than 1 cm, but these are likely to be evident on CT and they fall to about 40% for sub-centimetre lesions and even less in the presence of jaundice (Frohlich *et al.* 1999).

The addition of enhanced staging by laparoscopy has become standard practice in many centres for evaluation of the intra-abdominal contents. Even after good CT, further up-staging is seen in 10–20% of patients after laparoscopy. Resection rates of about 60% are usual in the pre-laparoscopic era. After the addition of laparoscopy in the staging paradigm, resection rates of 95% are more typical. The number of intent-to-cure resections performed is the same but the number of open-and-close cases is reduced to 5% or less. Subsequent addition of laparoscopic ultrasound has further increased the sensitivity for criteria of inoperability, especially for small liver metastases, small peritoneal metastases, evaluation of venous involvement and the retropancreatic region.

We have been keen proponents of laparoscopy and have shown our results using this strategy to yield about 95% accuracy in the prediction of operability through identification of patients with CT-occult criteria of irresectibility. The addition of laparoscopy to staging will re-assign about 30% of patients thought to be operative candidates at CT to being inoperable (Brooks *et al.* 2002; Elatar *et al.* 2003). As the sensitivity of extra-corporeal imaging rises then one might expect this number to fall. The Amsterdam group (Nieveen van Dijkum *et al.* 2002) have suggested that laparoscopy is unnecessary because it will not change the decision to operate on the basis that the best form of palliation is open bypass and so laparotomy will still be required. However, the detection rate of 'inoperable' features in this study was low (13%), in part because the study criteria only included histologically proven causes for inoperability. Had cases where vascular encasement or intrahepatic metastases were the causes for inoperability been included the detection rate would have doubled and be more in keeping with rates seen in other series of laparoscopy for pancreatic head tumours. Moreover, the inoperable cases were randomly assigned to endoscopic or surgical bypass. If a selective policy of surgical bypass in fit patients with only either nodal disease or vascular involvement as reasons for inoperability and endoscopic stenting reserved for the patients with liver or peritoneal metastases were to be implemented, then the benefits of laparoscopy are more obvious. Assuming the reason for inoperability is approximately equally divided between metastatic liver or peritoneal disease and local vascular or nodal disease, then the overall benefit in avoiding non-therapeutic laparotomy would be to about 15% of all patients considered for resection by CT and as many as 50% of patients considered inoperable at laparoscopy.

Only laparoscopy will identify patients with small liver or peritoneal deposits accurately, and it is precisely this group that have the most to lose from non-therapeutic laparotomy. Identification of this poorly performing group allows early endoscopic palliation and it is likely no further intervention will be required. The remainder are potential candidates for minimal access bypass surgery and may still avoid the need for laparotomy.

In our experience laparoscopy also adds useful subjective surgical information. The quality of the tissues, the texture of the pancreas and state of the vessels can be assessed. A short anaesthetic is helpful in evaluating the patient's ability to tolerate a larger procedure. All these factors add to the selection process. But taking into account the observations of the Dutch group we can plan three strategies for 'selection by laparoscopy'. Until extracorporeal imaging methods reach a high sensitivity for small volume disease in abdomen, we believe laparoscopy will continue to be of benefit in the selection process.

1. **Bypass in all patients not suitable for operation.**
   Using this strategy, unless the bypass is being performed laparoscopically, then all cases will come to laparotomy and so the value of laparoscopy is reduced to zero in avoiding laparotomy.

2. **Selective bypass, either elective or as required after stent failure or gastric obstruction.**
   In this setting. assuming that 50% of patients are likely to have vascular involvement/nodal disease as the cause of inoperability and predicted survival times of more than 6 months and that between 10% and 20% of these will develop gastric obstruction, then 10–15% of laparoscopically identified patients or about 3% of the total initially considered operable by CT will actually need an open operation for palliation. Indeed, these predicted figures are reproduced in the study from Espat et al. (1999) of 155 patients identified as inoperable at laparoscopy and are confirmed by Brooks in a later update (Brooks et al. 2002).

The remaining 97% will have either successful operation and resection, or are palliated without need for laparotomy.

3. **Totally endoscopic palliation for all inoperable patients.**
   Although the initial hospital stay is shorter for these patients, the total in-hospital time is longer. So this approach is only suitable for patients with a likely survival of less than 6 months either for medical and/or oncological reasons (Schwarz & Berger 2000).

Multivariate analysis shows that nodal disease, tumour differentiation and positive margins (R1 resection) at operation are independent predictors of poor outcome (Sperti 1997; Neoptolemos 2001). As surgeons we can only influence the last of these. There is no suggestion that extracorporeal imaging predicts for the ability to achieve negative margins. It is the retropancreatic margin that is most frequently positive (Luttges 1998) and whether any of the assessment tools contributes to the pre-operative assessment of oncologic integrity of the operation is doubtful. Laparoscopy with ultrasound allows us to look at the retropancreatic tissues closely. While accepting that this specific question has not been the subject of clinical trials, in our experience it has helped us to address this question. We believe this is reflected in our relatively low positive margin rate (Elatar *et al.* 2003).

The yield of peritoneal disease undetected (at CT) in body of pancreatic cancers is very high. These present with other symptoms, usually pain and weight loss, that is signs and symptoms of advanced disease, jaundice and obstruction are less common. Even fewer of these are operable and the patient very often deteriorates rapidly requiring urgent initiation of non-surgical support services. Laparoscopy rapidly identifies this group and allows gastric bypass, if required, without the requirement for open operation.

Conclusion

Pancreatic cancer carries a tumour-specific fatality of nearly 100%. The surgical challenge lies with rigorous selection of patients to undergo radical surgery to achieve R0 resection. Selection relates not only to evaluation of the feasibility of operation but the probability of oncologic benefit to the patient. Criteria that predicate for poor postoperative outcomes still need to be better defined. Currently accepted criteria should be sought and identified quickly such that these patients can be diverted to non-surgical pathways. No single examination successfully answers all of the questions. The superiority of MRI in contrast resolution makes it useful in lesions of unknown aetiology, for example with a major inflammatory component but does not supersede CT scan in staging. Small lesions or strong clinical suspicion in the absence of a mass lesion are probably best investigated by EUS. For the present, PET scanning shows no advantage in diagnosis but may be of value in evaluation of potential metastatic disease such as distant nodes and extra-abdominal sites of metastases. Angiography is no longer considered as necessary. Dual-phase spiral CT scan provides good contrast and spatial resolution making it the 'workhorse' of diagnosis and staging and will in time be replaced by multislice CT. The successive improvements in CT have shone the light on diagnosis, evaluation of the vessels in particular and to some extent the liver (Clarke *et al.* 2003). However, examination to fully qualify the abdomen and identify small hepatic and peritoneal metastases, too small to be detected on CT, is best achieved by laparoscopy. Moreover, laparoscopy allows segregation of inoperable patients into those best palliated by endoscopy from those likely to benefit from surgical bypass. The potential for minimal access bypass exists if required at staging laparoscopy. About 15% of patients should be spared unhelpful laparotomy by this strategy. Whether laparoscopic evaluation with ultrasound of the retroperitoneum or intraportal ultrasound enhances the negative margin rate is an unanswered question; we are attempting to address this issue in our own practice. Our management paradigm is shown in Figure 9.1 and reflects these ideas.

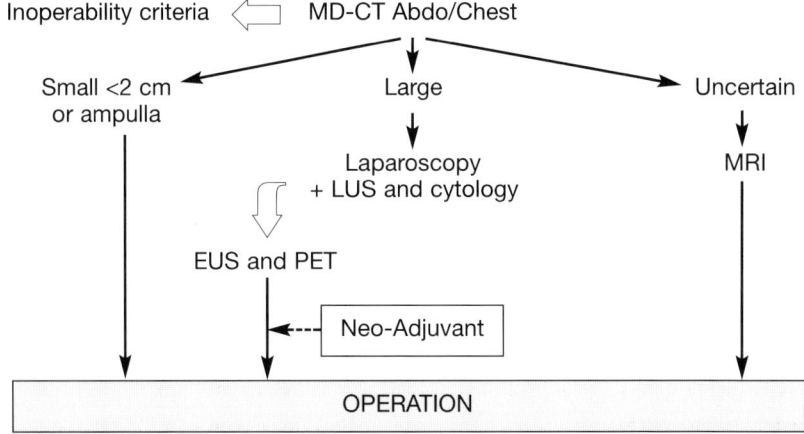

Figure 9.1 Management pathway for periampullary mass suspected to be cancer.

References

Barkin, J. S., Goldberg, R. I., Sfakianakis, G. N. & Levi, J. (1986). Pancreatic carcinoma is associated with delayed gastric emptying. *Digestive Diseases and Sciences* **31**, 265–267.

Barreiro, C. J., Lillemoe, K. D., Koniaris, L. G. *et al.* (2002). Diagnostic laparoscopy for periampullary and pancreatic cancer: what is the true benefit? *Journal of Gastrointestinal Surgery* **6**, 75–81.

Brooks, A. D., Mallis, M. J., Brennan, M. F. *et al.* (2002). The value of laparoscopy in the management of ampullary, duodenal, and distal bile duct tumors. *Journal of Gastrointestinal Surgery* **6**, 139–145.

Cannon, M. E., Carpenter, S. L., Elta, G. H. *et al.* (1999). EUS compared with CT, magnetic resonance imaging, and angiography and the influence of biliary stenting on staging accuracy of ampullary neoplasms. *Gastrointestinal Endoscopy* **50**, 27–33.

Clarke, D. L., Thomson, S. R., Madiba, T. E. *et al.* (2003). Preoperative imaging of pancreatic cancer: a management-orientated approach. *Journal of the American College of Surgeons* **196**, 119–129.

Del Frate, C., Zanardi, R., Mortele, K. *et al.* (2002). Advances in imaging for pancreatic disease. *Current Gastroenterology Reports* **4**, 140–148.

Diederichs, C. G., Staib, L., Vogel, J. *et al.* (2000). Values and limitations of 18F-fluorodeoxyglucose-positron-emission tomography with preoperative evaluation of patients with pancreatic masses. *Pancreas* **20**, 109–116.

Diehl, S. J., Lachmann, K. J., Sadick, M. *et al.* (1998). Pancreatic cancer: value of dual-phase helical CT scan in assessing respectability. *Radiology* **206**, 373–378.

DiMagno, E. P., Reber, H. A. & Tempero, M. A. (1999). AGA technical review on the epidemiology, diagnosis, and treatment of pancreatic ductal adenocarcinoma. American Gastroenterological Association. *Gastroenterology* **117**, 1464–1484.

Elatar, A., Durkin, D., Sweeney, T. J. *et al.* (2003). Laparoscopic staging predictability of curative resection in pancreatic head tumours. *Surgical Endoscopy and Other Interventional Techniques* **17** (Suppl.), 77.

Espat, N. J., Brennan, M. F. & Conlon, K. C. (1999). Patients with laparoscopically staged unresectable pancreatic cancer do not require subsequent surgical biliary or gastric bypass. *Journal of the American College of Surgeons* **188**, 649–655.

Everhart, J. & Wright, D. (1995). Diabetes mellitus as a risk factor for pancreatic cancer. A meta-analysis. *Journal of the American Medical Association* **273**, 1605–1609.

Frohlich, A., Diederichs, C. G., Staib, L. *et al.* (1999). Detection of liver metastases from pancreatic cancer using FDG PET. *Journal of Nuclear Medicine* **40**, 250–255.

Fujino, Y., Suzuki, Y., Ajiki, T. *et al.* (2003). Predicting factors for survival of patients with unresectable pancreatic cancer: a management guideline. *Hepatogastroenterology* **50**, 250–253.

Fong, Y., Blumgart, L. H., Fortner, J. G. *et al.* (1995). Pancreatic or liver resection for malignancy is safe and effective for the elderly. *Annals of Surgery* **222**, 426–434.

Gold, E. B. & Goldin, S. B. (1998). Epidemiology of and risk factors for pancreatic cancer. *Surgical Oncology Clinics of North America* **7**, 67–91.

Hahn, M. & Faigel, D. O. (2001). Frequency of mediastinal lymph node metastases in patients undergoing EUS evaluation of pancreaticobiliary masses. *Gastrointestinal Endoscopy* **54**, 331–335.

Harrison, L. E. & Brennan, M. F. (1998). Portal vein resection for pancreatic adenocarcinoma. *Surgical Oncology Clinics of North America* **7**, 165–181.

Hewitt, P. M., Beningfield, S. J., Bornman, P. C. *et al.* (1998). Pancreatic carcinoma. Diagnostic and prognostic implications of a normal pancreatogram. *Surgical Endoscopy* **12**, 867–869.

Horton, K. M. (2002). Multidetector CT and three-dimensional imaging of the pancreas: state of the art. *Journal of Gastrointestinal Surgery* **6**, 126–128.

Huguier, M. & Mason, N. P. (1999). Treatment of cancer of the exocrine pancreas. *American Journal of Surgery* **177**, 257–265.

Janes, R. H. Jr, Niederhuber, J. E., Chmiel, J. S. *et al.* (1996). National patterns of care for pancreatic cancer. Results of a survey by the Commission on Cancer. *Annals of Surgery* **223**, 261–272.

Jimenez, R. E., Warshaw, A. L., Rattner, D. W. *et al.* (2000). Impact of laparoscopic staging in the treatment of pancreatic cancer. *Archives of Surgery* **135**, 409–414.

Jurowich, C., Meyer, W., Adamus, R. *et al.* (2000). Portal vein resection in the framework of surgical therapy of pancreatic head carcinoma: clarification of indication by improved preoperative diagnostic procedures? *Chirug* **71**, 803–807.

Kalady, M. F., Clary, B. M., Clark, L. A. *et al.* (2002) Clinical utility of positron emission tomography in the diagnosis and management of periampullary neoplasms. *Annals of Surgical Oncology* **9**, 799–806.

Kalser, M. H., Barkin, J. & MacIntyre, J. M. (1985) Pancreatic cancer. Assessment of prognosis by clinical presentation. *Cancer* **56**, 397–402.

Kaneko, T., Nakano, A. & Takagi, H. (1998). Intraportal endovascular ultrasonography for pancreatic cancer. *Seminars in Surgical Oncology* **15**, 47–51.

Kelsen, D. P., Portenoy, R., Thaler, H. *et al.* (1997). Pain as a predictor of outcome in patients with operable pancreatic carcinoma. *Surgery* **122**, 53–59.

Kotwall, C. A., Maxwell, J. G., Brinker, C. C. *et al.* (2002). National Estimates of mortality rates for radical pancreaticoduodenectomy in 25,000 patients. *Annals of Surgical Oncology* **9**, 847–854.

Legmann, P., Vignaux, O., Dousset, B. *et al.* (1998). Pancreatic tumors: comparison of dual-phase helical CT and endoscopic sonography. *American Journal of Roentgenology* **170**, 1315–1322.

Lei, S., Kini, J., Kim, K. & Howard, J. M. (1994). Pancreatic cancer. Cytologic study of peritoneal washings. *Archives of Surgery* **129**, 639–642.

Luque-de León, E., Tsiotos, G. G., Balsiger, B. *et al.* (1999). Staging laparoscopy for pancreatic cancer should be used to select the best means of palliation and not only to maximize the resectability rate. *Journal of Gastrointestinal Surgery* **3**, 111–118.

Luttges, J., Vogel, I., Menke, M. *et al.* (1998). The retroperitoneal resection margin and vessel involvement are important factors determining survival after pancreaticoduodenectomy for ductal adenocarcinoma of the head of the pancreas. *Virchows Archiv* **433**, 237–242.

Mann, D. V., Edwards, R., Ho, S. *et al.* (2000). Elevated tumour marker CA19-9: clinical interpretation and influence of obstructive jaundice. *European Journal of Surgical Oncology* **26**, 474–479.

McCarthy, M. J., Evans, J., Sagar, G. *et al.* (1998). Prediction of resectability of pancreatic malignancy by computed tomography. *British Journal of Surgery* **85**, 320–325.

Midwinter, M. J., Beveridge, C. J., Wilsdon, J. B. *et al.* (1999). Correlation between spiral computed tomography, endoscopic ultrasonography and findings at operation in pancreatic and ampullary tumours. *British Journal of Surgery* **86**, 189–193.

Neoptolemos, J. P., Stocken, D. D., Dunn J. A. *et al.* (2001). Influence of resection margins on survival for patients with pancreatic cancer treated by adjuvant chemoradiation and/or chemotherapy in the ESPAC-1 randomized controlled trial. *Annals of Surgery* **234**, 758–768.

Nieveen van Dijkum, E. J., Romijn, M. G., Terwee, C. B. *et al.* (2003). Laparoscopic staging and subsequent palliation in patients with peripancreatic carcinoma. *Annals of Surgery* **237**, 66–73.

Povoski, S. P., Karpeh, M. S. Jr, Conlon, K. C. *et al.* (1999). Preoperative biliary drainage: impact on intraoperative bile cultures and infectious morbidity and mortality after pancreaticoduodenectomy. *Journal of Gastrointestinal Surgery* **3**, 496–505.

Reber, H. A. & Gloor, B. (1998). Radical pancreatectomy. *Surgical Oncology Clinics of North America* **7**, 157–163.

Rickles, F. R. & Edwards, R. L. (1983). Activation of blood coagulation in cancer: Trousseau's syndrome revisited. *Blood* **62**, 14–31.

Rosch, T., Dittler, H. J., Strobel, K. *et al.* (2000). Endoscopic ultrasound criteria for vascular invasion in the staging of cancer of the head of the pancreas: a blind reevaluation of videotapes. *Gastrointestinal Endoscopy* **52**, 469–477.

Sahani, D., Prasad, S., Saini, S. *et al.* (2002). Cystic pancreatic neoplasms evaluation by CT and magnetic resonance cholangiopancreatography. *Gastrointestinal Endoscopy Clinics of North America* **12**, 657–672.

Schwarz, A. & Beger, H. G. (2000). Biliary and gastric bypass or stenting in non-resectable periampullary cancer: analysis on the basis of controlled trials. *International Journal of Pancreatology* **27**, 51–58.

Schwarz, M., Pauls, S., Sokiranski, R. *et al.* (2001). Is a preoperative multidiagnostic approach to predict resectability of periampullary tumours still effective? *American Journal of Surgery* **182**, 243–249.

Shibata, C., Kobari, M., Tsuchiya, T. *et al.* (2001). Pancreatectomy combined with superior mesenteric-portal vein resection for adenocarcinoma in pancreas. *World Journal of Surgery* **25**, 1002–1005.

Sindelar, W. F. (1989). Clinical experience with regional pancreatectomy for adenocarcinoma of the pancreas. *Archives of Surgery* **124**, 127–132.

Spencer, M. P., Sarr, M. G. & Nagorney, D. M. (1990). Radical pancreatectomy for pancreatic cancer in the elderly. Is it safe and justified? *Annals of Surgery* **212**, 140–143.

Sperti, C., Pasquali, C., Piccoli, A. *et al.* (1997). Recurrence after resection for ductal adenocarcinoma of the pancreas. *World Journal of Surgery* **21**, 195–200.

Trede, M., Rumstadt, B. & Wendl, K. *et al.* (1997). Ultrafast magnetic resonance imaging improves the staging of pancreatic tumors. *Annals of Surgery* **226**, 393–405.

Valinas, R., Barrier, A., Montravers, F. *et al.* (2002). 18 F-fluorodeoxyglucose positron emission tomography for characterization and initial staging of pancreatic tumors. [In French.] *Gastroenterologie Clinique et Biologie* **26**, 888–892.

Chapter 10

Advanced pancreatic cancer: the case for chemotherapy

Russell D. Petty and Marianne C. Nicolson

Introduction

The treatment of advanced pancreatic carcinoma represents a formidable challenge. The natural history and clinical features of the disease mark it as one of the most aggressive human cancers, and result in most patients presenting with advanced disease. In the UK, 7000 new cases are diagnosed annually and 5500 present with advanced disease (GLOBOCAN 2000).

The median survival of untreated patients with advanced pancreatic cancer is poor (3–4 months) but, in addition, disease-related symptoms such as pain, obstructive jaundice, fatigue, anorexia and gastric outlet obstruction result in a complex clinical syndrome with considerable morbidity. The importance of control of these symptoms is clear, but has only relatively recently been addressed in clinical trials of systemic chemotherapy. In these trials, measures such as symptom palliation and quality of life have been evaluated, as well as the more traditional end-points of response rates, progression-free and overall survival. Well-designed clinical investigations of this type have shown that systemic chemotherapy confers benefits in symptom control and quality of life (Nicolson *et al.* 1995; Carmichael *et al.* 1996; Burris *et al.* 1997; Berlin *et al.* 2002; Colucci *et al.* 2002; Louvet *et al.* 2002; Rocha Lima *et al.* 2002; Scheithauer *et al.* 2003; Stathopoulos *et al.* 2003). These benefits are conferred in addition to the supportive care provided by surgery, interventional radiology and palliative medicine, each of which have made considerable progress in their own right. The design and validation of novel efficacy end-points such as clinical benefit response (CBR) has been critical in this work, and when analysed in these terms the clinical trial data provide good evidence and clear guidelines for the use of chemotherapy in advanced pancreatic carcinoma.

The challenges

There are several challenges that can be identified and that need to be addressed in the clinical use of chemotherapy in advanced pancreatic carcinoma. These issues are also relevant to the design and execution of clinical trials in this area, and applicable to much-needed translational research.

Patient fitness

The need to balance the efficacy and toxicity of therapy is central to the management of all cancers, but is particularly pertinent in the management of advanced pancreatic cancer. Here, the prognosis and already considerable co-existent morbidity due to disease-related symptoms (present in many patients at diagnosis) mean that anything more than the mildest of treatment-related toxicity is unacceptable. This is an important issue not only for evaluation of therapies but also for patient selection for systemic chemotherapy. The identification of individual patients who are most likely to benefit from particular therapies is a major challenge for translational research in all malignancies, but for reasons of patient fitness is particularly important for advanced pancreatic cancer.

Histological confirmation

Whereas histological diagnosis is ideally an essential part of the management of advanced pancreatic carcinoma, in practice even under the most optimal circumstances this is not always possible (Petty *et al.* 2003). Technical issues aside, in this group of patients with difficult symptom control problems and poor prognosis, it is often not appropriate to make multiple attempts at biopsy. However, clinical experience and published reviews of cases without a histological diagnosis do suggest that misdiagnosis is rare after careful review of the clinical and radiological features of individual cases in the multidisciplinary setting (Bottger *et al.* 1999). This is certainly an issue in routine clinical practice, but is also important for the pragmatic design of clinical trials and highly relevant to translational research, where the provision of clinical tissue specimens is vital.

Baseline measurements and objective response evaluation

The problems associated with the radiological assessment of objective response in pancreatic cancer are well documented (Ballard *et al.* 1995). In particular, the often intense desmoplastic reaction associated with the primary tumour can make measurement difficult and subjective. The independent review of radiology in clinical trials has addressed this issue to some extent; however, it remains an important issue in clinical practice. In addition, the presence of tumours composed of a minority of malignant cells and a majority of inflammatory and stromal cells presents further problems for objective response assessment. This can present difficulties in clinical trials of newer biological and targeted agents, many of which appear to be more cytostatic than cytotoxic. Accordingly, although objective response remains important, it is clear that it must be interpreted in the context of other efficacy measurements as determined by other clinical trial end-points.

End-points

The use of composite end-points such as CBR, involving measurements of pain, Karnofsky performance status and weight, have revealed that up to 60% of patients with advanced pancreatic cancer may benefit from chemotherapy (Berlin *et al*. 2002; Colucci *et al*. 2002; Louvet *et al.* 2002; Scheithauer *et al.* 2003; Stathopoulos *et al.* 2003). For a positive CBR, a patient must experience 4 weeks of improvement in at least one of the components of CBR without any deterioration in the others. The strength of such measures lies in their relevance to the clinical management of the symptom control problems presented in advanced pancreatic carcinoma. The benefit achieved by the successful management of these symptoms is clear, but also demonstrated by concurrent quality-of-life assessments. As we will discuss, the design of further novel clinical efficacy measurements in the era of combination chemotherapy and targeted therapies remains an ongoing challenge for clinical researchers in advanced pancreatic cancer.

Clinical trials of chemotherapy in advanced pancreatic cancer

Chemotherapy versus best supportive care

A recent meta-analysis identified nine trials of chemotherapy versus best supportive care (BSC) involving over 600 patients, in advanced pancreatic carcinoma (Fung *et al*. 2003). All used 5-fluorouracil (5-FU)-based combination chemotherapy and although symptom control was not universally assessed, all demonstrate a survival benefit. Where symptom control was assessed, chemotherapy was found to be of additional benefit (Fung *et al*. 2003). Although the precise nature and definition of BSC applied in several of these studies might be debated (especially by today's standards), the efficacy and feasibility of the use of systemic chemotherapy in advanced pancreatic cancer is demonstrated. The main contribution of these early studies has been as a catalyst to promote more extensive evaluation of systemic chemotherapy in advanced pancreatic carcinoma.

Single-agent chemotherapy

A wide variety of single agents have been investigated in advanced pancreatic carcinoma. Often, high response rates and efficacy have been suggested in phase II trials but have not been seen in phase III investigations. This raises important issues of patient selection for systemic therapy. It is clear that many cytotoxics have efficacy, but the phase III trial of gemcitabine versus 5-FU monotherapy performed by Burris *et al*. (1997) was the first to formally assess symptom control issues, and in doing so has established a standard of investigation and evaluation that other agents must be tested against. In this study, 126 chemotherapy-naive patients were randomised to receive either 5-FU (600 mg/m^2 i.v. bolus weekly for 7 out of 8 weeks, then 3 from 4 weeks thereafter) or gemcitabine (1000 mg/m^2, i.v. bolus weekly for 7 out of 8weeks, then 3 from 4 weeks thereafter). CBR was seen in 23.8% of patients receiving gemcitabine compared with 5% receiving 5-FU ($p = 0.0022$). In addition, the median time to progression was significantly longer for gemcitabine (9 weeks versus 4 weeks for 5-FU, $p = 0.002$) and there was a small but significant survival advantage for gemcitabine (5.65 months versus 4.41 months, $p = 0.0025$). The response rates for gemcitabine and 5-FU were not significantly different (5.4% for gemcitabine, 0% for 5-FU). This illustrates that response rate is not necessarily a useful endpoint for demonstrating the efficacy of chemotherapy in advanced pancreatic cancer. As a consequence of this study, single-agent gemcitabine is considered the 'gold standard' by many for systemic treatment for patients with advanced pancreatic cancer.

A recent phase II study has suggested that the scheduling of gemcitabine may be important. Pharmacokinetic investigation has shown that the active metabolite of gemcitabine (gemcitabine triphosphate) is accumulated more effectively by longer infusion times and therefore shorter infusions may be less effective. Tempero *et al.* (2003) randomised 92 patients with locally advanced or metastatic pancreatic carcinoma to a dose intense treatment of gemcitabine (2200 mg/m^2 as a 30 minute infusion, typically standard infusion time) or to a fixed dose rate (FDR) treatment with 1500 mg/m^2 given at a rate of 10 mg/m^2/minute (both weekly for 3 out of 4 weeks). The median survival for all patients was improved with FDR treatment (8.0 months versus 5.0 months, $p = 0.013$). The 1- and 2-year survival rates for all patients were also significantly better for FDR treatment (1-year survival 28.8% versus 9%, $p = 0.014$, and 2-year survival 18.3% versus 2.2% , $p = 0.007$). Patients in the FDR infusion arm experienced consistently more haematological toxicity. Pharmacokinetic analyses demonstrated a twofold increase in intracellular gemcitabine triphosphate concentration in the FDR arm ($p = 0.046$). The FDR treatment strategy is currently under evaluation in an Eastern Co-operative Oncology Group phase III trial.

Combination chemotherapy

Several both gemcitabine- and non-gemcitabine-based combination chemotherapy regimens have been evaluated in both phase II and phase III trials (Nicolson *et al.* 1995; Reni *et al.* 2001; Stathopoulos *et al.* 2001, 2003; Berlin *et al.* 2002; Colucci *et al.* 2002; Kindler *et al.* 2002; Louvet *et al.* 2002; Rocha Lima *et al.* 2002; Ryan *et al.* 2002; Scheithauer *et al.* 2003; Petty *et al.* 2003). Several non-gemcitabine-based combinations, for example mitomycin C, cisplatin and 5-FU (MCF), have demonstrated efficacy and tolerability (Petty *et al.* 2003). However, given the good symptom control and quality-of-life data that exist for gemcitabine, combined with its ease of administration and good toxicity profile, many authors consider only gemcitabine-based combinations as worthy of further investigation. The results of studies with gemcitabine-based combination chemotherapy are summarised in Table 10.1. Again, although phase II studies have often been encouraging, the results overall from phase III trials of combination chemotherapy versus single-agent gemcitabine

Table 10.1 Summary of key studies with gemcitabine-based combination chemotherapy in advanced pancreatic carcinoma. This is not a comprehensive list of studies; studies selected are representative of those performed for each regimen. Although there is no overall consistent clinical benefit for combination chemotherapy, a consistent finding is that some measures of clinical efficacy are promising whereas others are not. This illustrates the complex risk–benefit analysis that is required and which current trials have not fully resolved. More details and discussion in the text.

Regimen	Study	Phase	Number of patients	Stage III/IV	RR (%)	TTP (months)	MS (months) (%)	1-year survival (%)	2-year survival	CBR (%)
Gemcitabine plus 5-FU	Gem/5FU versus Gem (Berlin et al. 2002)	III	162	17/145	6.9	3.4	6.7	NG	NG	NG
			160	16/144	5.6 (ns)	2.2 (ns)	5.4(ns)	NG	NG	NG
Gemcitabine plus capecitabine	Gem/Cap versus Gem (Scheithauer et al. 2003)	II	42	0/42	17	5.1	9.5	31.8	NG	48
			41	0/41	14 (ns)	4.0 (ns)	8.2 (ns)	37.2 (ns)	NG	33 (ns)
Gemcitabine plus cisplatin	Gem/Cis versus Gem (Colucci et al. 2002)	II	43	10/33	26	2	7.5	11	NG	52
			43	14/29	9 ($p = 0.02^*$)	5 ($p=0.04^*$)	4.5 (ns)	11 (ns)	NG	49 (ns)
Gemcitabine plus irinotecan	Gem/IRN (Rocha Lima et al. 2002)	II	45	13/32	20	2.8	5.7	27	NG	NG
Gemcitabine plus docetaxel	Gem/Doc (Stathopoulos et al. 2001)	II	54	16/38	13	7.0	8.0	22.5	NG	78
	Gem/Doc (Ryan et al. 2002)	II	34	0/34	18	3.8	8.9	29	NG	NG
Gemcitabine plus oxaliplatin	Gem/Ox (Louvet et al. 2002)	II	64	30/34	30.6	5.3	9.2	36	NG	40
Gemcitabine plus pemetrexed	Gem/Pem (Kindler et al. 2002)	II	42	2/40	15	NG	6.5	29	NG	NG

RR, response rate; NG, not given; (ns), not significant ($p > 0.05$); Gem=gemcitabine; 5-FU, 5-fluorouracil; Cap, capecitabine; Cis, cisplatin; Doc, docetaxel; Irn, irinotecan; Ox, oxaliplatin; Pem, pemetrexed.

have been disappointing and have not shown a consistent, clinically significant benefit for combination chemotherapy (Nicolson *et al.* 1995; Reni *et al.* 2001; Stathopoulos *et al.* 2001, 2003; Berlin *et al.* 2002, Colucci *et al.* 2002; Kindler *et al.* 2002; Louvet *et al.* 2002; Rocha Lima *et al.* 2002, Ryan *et al.* 2002; Petty *et al.* 2003; Scheithauer *et al.* 2003). However, caution must be taken with the interpretation of current clinical trial data in this regard, particularly when assessing additional efficacy against increased toxicity of combination therapy. As already discussed, CBR and quality-of-life measurements must be carefully evaluated as well as more traditional methods of response and success of treatment. Accordingly, in many phase III studies, some outcomes appear to offer encouragement but others are negative. The result is a complex risk–benefit analysis that current trials have not always addressed or fully resolved. While studies are ongoing (phase III trials for single-agent gemcitabine versus combinations of gemcitabine/capecitabine, gemcitabine/oxaliplatin, gemcitabine/cisplatin, gemcitabine/irinotecan, gemcitabine/docetaxel and gemcitabine/pemetrexed are ongoing), new measures to assess treatment efficacy are needed and will prove to be of particular value in the assessment of novel and targeted agents.

Novel and targeted agents

Several novel and targeted agents have been evaluated in advanced pancreatic cancer, including matrix metalloproteinase inhibitors (MMPIs), farnesyltransferase inhibitors, and agents directed against epidermal growth factor receptor (EGFR) or vascular epidermal growth factor (VEGFR) signalling. Phase I and II trials have demonstrated the safety, good toxicity profiles and activity of these agents in advanced pancreatic cancer, but overall the efficacy results have been disappointing so far (Abbruzzese *et al.* 2001; Hidalgo *et al.* 2001; Bramhall *et al.* 2001, 2002; Cohen *et al.* 2003; Kindler *et al.* 2003). Superiority to single-agent gemcitabine had not been demonstrated in most cases until the advent of the PA3 trial which shows significant survival benefit from the addition of erlotinib to standard gemcitabine therapy (Abbruzzese *et al.* 2001; Bramhall *et al.* 2001; Hidalgo *et al.* 2001; Kindler *et al.* 2003). However, like other malignancies, the real challenge with these agents is the design of the clinical trials, and the identification of particular patients who might benefit most from their use. This latter point addresses the issue of how best to integrate novel targeted therapies with current cytotoxics and also the issue of individualisation of therapy for patients. This will require novel diagnostic approaches that will identify the presence or absence of the target and the probability of success in individual patients. Global tumour profiling technologies either at the genomic, transcriptomic or proteomic level are currently addressing this, and the integration of the results of such translational research into clinical trial design and ultimately into clinical practice will provide a considerable challenge.

Overall, agents that inhibit the EGFR and VEGFR signalling pathways look the most promising (Baker *et al.* 2002; Xiong *et al.* 2002). This promise has already been fulfilled in the case of the small molecule EGFR tyrosine kinase inhibitor, erlotinib. In the PA3 trial conducted by the National Cancer Institute of Canada patients with inoperable pancreatic cancer receiving standard gemcitabine therapy were randomised to additional treatment with erlotinib 100 mg/day or placebo. Overall survival was significantly increased (by 23% $p = 0.025$) as was progression-free survival and the percentage of patients alive at one year (24% versus 17%) in the erlotinib arm (Moore *et al.* 2005). A phase III trial of the anti-EGFR monoclonal antibody cetuximab in combination with gemcitabine is currently ongoing (Baker *et al.* 2002; Xiong *et al.* 2002). However, it is clear that more translational research is needed to identify additional novel targets.

Second-line therapy

Effective second-line therapies are available for patients with advanced pancreatic cancer. For those patients previously treated with 5-FU-based therapies, gemcitabine is an effective second-line therapy. A phase II study and a retrospective analysis of 982 patients treated on an investigational new drug programme with single-agent gemcitabine after first-line 5-FU-based therapy suggests that symptomatic response can be achieved in 18–27%, and objective response in 10.5–12% (Rothenberg *et al.* 1996; Storniolo *et al.* 1999). Stable disease was seen in a further 29.8% of patients in the phase II study (Rotenberg *et al.* 1996). The median time to progression and median survivals reported were 2.5 and 2.7 months, and 3.9 and 4.8 months, respectively. These figures illustrate the poor prognosis in this group of patients with refractory disease, but it is clear that symptomatic improvement and significant disease control can be achieved in a clinically relevant proportion of patients without undue toxicity.

For those patients who have received gemcitabine first line, irinotecan may represent an effective second-line therapy; however, concerns about toxicity in this vunerable group of patients remain. In a phase II study ($n = 31$) , patients received gemcitabine, 5-FU/FA and cisplatin followed by irinotecan (80 mg/m^2 repeated every 2 weeks); the median time to progressive disease was reported as 10 weeks and median survival 11.8 months (Araneo *et al.* 2003).

Conclusions

The treatment of advanced pancreatic cancer with chemotherapy provides several challenges unique to this disease. The establishment of single-agent gemcitabine as the 'gold standard' has required the creation and evaluation of novel clinical efficacy measurements. In doing so, it has provided unequivocal evidence for the benefit of systemic chemotherapy in advanced pancreatic cancer. Combination chemotherapy with gemcitabine has greater toxicity, but so far has not consistently been shown to be of improved efficacy. However, evaluation of any additional benefit against additional toxicity in this group of patients is a complex issue, which has not been completely resolved in current trials and will most likely require additional clinical efficacy measurements. The evaluation of novel targeted agents is likewise incomplete and will require innovative clinical trial design. Early results (for example with MMPIs and farnesyltransferase inhibitors) have not shown superiority to single-agent gemcitabine or additional benefit in combination. However, phase II data with agents targeting EGFR signalling are more promising, and phase III trials of combination therapy with gemcitabine are underway. The increasing number of agents that appear to have efficacy in advanced pancreatic cancer is providing the opportunity for the evaluation of second-line therapies. Data are emerging to suggest the potential for several strategies here.

Overall, chemotherapy is of established benefit for advanced pancreatic cancer but the future will involve the realisation of two interrelated aims. Firstly, the identification of novel targets and new agents in translational research, and secondly the optimisation of the use of targeted agents and conventional cytotoxics in individual patients. In both regards the use of global microarray profiling technologies holds considerable (albeit as yet unproven) promise. However, the integration of such technologies into clinical trial design and into clinical practice will provide a significant challenge.

References

Abbruzzese, J. L., Rosenberg, A., Xiong, Q., LoBuglio, A., Schmidt, W. A., Wolff, R., Needle, M. H. & Waksa, H. (2001). Phase II study of anti-epidermal growth factor receptor (EGFR) antibody cetuximab (IMC-C225) in combination with gemcitabine in patients with advanced pancreatic cancer. *Proceedings of the American Society of Clinical Oncology* **20**, 130.

Araneo, M., Bruckner, H. W., Grossbard M. L., Frager, D., Homel, P., Marino, J. *et al.* (2003). Biweekly low-dose sequential gemcitabine, 5-fluorouracil, leucovorin, and cisplatin (GFP): a highly active novel therapy for metastatic adenocarcinoma of the exocrine pancreas. *Cancer Investigation* **21**, 489–496.

Baker, C. H., Solorzano, C. C. & Fidler, I. J. (2002). Blockade of vascular endothelial growth factor receptor and epidermal growth factor receptor signaling for therapy of metastatic human pancreatic cancer. *Cancer Research* **62**, 1996–2003.

Ballard, R. B., Hoffman, J. P., Guttman, M. C. *et al.* (1995). How accurate is size measurement of pancreas cancer masses by computed axial tomography (CT) scanning? *American Surgeon* **61**, 686–691.

Berlin, J. D., Catalano, P., Thomas, J. P., Kugler, J. W., Haller, D. G. & Benson, A. B. III. (2002). Phase III study of gemcitabine in combination with fluorouracil versus gemcitabine alone in patients with advanced pancreatic carcinoma: Eastern Cooperative Oncology Group Trial E2297. *Journal of Clinical Oncology* **20**, 3270–3275.

Bottger, T. C. & Junginger, T. (1999). Treatment of tumors of the pancreatic head with suspected but unproved malignancy: is a nihilistic approach justified? *World Journal of Surgery* **23**, 158–162.

Bramhall, S. R., Rosemurgy, A., Brown, P. D., Bowry, C. & Buckels, J. A. (2001). Marimastat as first-line therapy for patients with unresectable pancreatic cancer: a randomized trial. *Journal of Clinical Oncology* **19**, 3447–3455.

Bramhall, S. R., Schulz, J., Nemunaitis, J., Brown, P. D., Baillet, M. & Buckels, J. A. (2002). A double-blind placebo-controlled, randomised study comparing gemcitabine and marimastat with gemcitabine and placebo as first line therapy in patients with advanced pancreatic cancer. *British Journal of Cancer* **87**, 161–167.

Burris, H. A., Moore, M. J., Anderson, J., Green, M. R., Rothenberg, M. L., Modiano, M. R. *et al.* (1997). Improvements in survival and clinical benefit with gemcitabine as first-line therapy for patients with advanced pancreas cancer: a randomised trial. *Journal of Clinical Oncology* **15**, 2403–2413.

Carmichael, J., Fink, U., Russell, R. C., Spittle, M. F., Harris, A. L., Spiessi, G. *et al.* (1996). Phase II study of gemcitabine in patients with advanced pancreatic cancer. *British Journal of Cancer* **73**, 101–105.

Cohen, S. J., Ho, L., Ranganathan, S., Abbruzzese, J. L., Alpaugh, R. K., Beard, M. *et al.* (2003). Phase II and pharmacodynamic study of the farnesyltransferase inhibitor R115777 as initial therapy in patients with metastatic pancreatic adenocarcinoma. *Journal of Clinical Oncology* **21**, 1301–1306.

Colucci, G., Giuliani, F., Gebbia, V., Biglietto, M., Rabitti, P., Uomo, G. *et al.* (2002). Gemcitabine alone or with cisplatin for the treatment of patients with locally advanced and/or metastatic pancreatic carcinoma: a prospective, randomized phase III study of the Gruppo Oncologia dell'Italia Meridionale. *Cancer* **94**, 902–910.

Fung, M. C., Ishiguro, S., Takayama, S., Morizane, T., Adachi, S. & Sakata, T. (2003). Survival benefit of chemotherapy treatment in advanced pancreatic cancer: a meta-analysis. *Proceedings of the American Society of Clinical Oncology* **22**, 288 (abstract 1155).

GLOBOCAN (2000). *Cancer Incidence. Mortality and Prevalence Worldwide, version 1.0.* IARC Cancerbase no. 5. Lyon, France: IARC Press. Available at http://www-dep.iarc.fr/globocan/globocan.htm

Hidalgo, M., Siu, L. L., Nemunaitis, J., Rizzo, J., Hammond, L. A., Takimoto, C. *et al.* (2001). Phase I and pharmacologic study of OSI-774, an epidermal growth factor receptor tyrosine kinase inhibitor, in patients with advanced solid malignancies. *Journal of Clinical Oncology* **19**, 3267–3279.

Kindler, H. L. (2002). The pemetrexed/gemcitabine combination in pancreatic cancer. *Cancer* **95**(4 Suppl.), 928–932.

Kindler, H. L., Ansari, R., Lester, E., Locker, G., Nattam, S., Stadler, W. M., Wade-Oliver, K. & Vokes, E. E. (2003). Bevacizumab (B) plus gemcitabine (G) in patients (pts) with advanced pancreatic cancer (PC). *Proceedings of the American Society of Clinical Oncology* **22**, 259.

Louvet, C., Andre, T., Lledo, G., Hammel, P., Bleiberg, H., Bouleuc, C. *et al.* (2002). Gemcitabine combined with oxaliplatin in advanced pancreatic adenocarcinoma: final results of a GERCOR multicenter phase II study. *Journal of Clinical Oncology* **20**, 1512–1518.

Moore, M. J., Goldstein, D., Hamm, J. *et al.* (2005). A phase III double blind trial of gemcitabine +/- erlotinib in locally advanced/metastatic pancreatic carcinoma. *Proceedings of the American Society of Clinical Oncology* GI Cancer Symposium. Abstract 77.

Nicolson, M., Webb, A., Cunningham, D., Norman, A., O'Brien, M., Hill, A. *et al.* (1995). Cisplatin and protracted venous infusion 5-fluorouracil (CF) – good symptom relief with low toxicity in advanced pancreatic carcinoma. *Annals of Oncology* **6**, 801–804.

Petty, R., Nicolson, M. C., Skaria, S., Sinclair, T. S., Samuel, L. M. & Koruth, M. A (2003). A phase II study of mitomycin C, cisplatin and protracted infusional 5-fluorouracil in advanced pancreatic carcinoma: efficacy and low toxicity. *Annals of Oncology* **14**, 1100–1105.

Reni, M., Passoni, P., Panucci, M. G., Nicoletti, R., Galli, L., Balzano, G. *et al.* (2001). Definitive results of a phase II trial of cisplatin, epirubicin, continuous-infusion fluorouracil, and gemcitabine in stage IV pancreatic adenocarcinoma. *Journal of Clinical Oncology* **19**, 2679–2686.

Rocha Lima, C. M., Savarese, D., Bruckner, H., Dudek, A., Eckardt, J., Hainsworth, J. *et al.* (2002). Irinotecan plus gemcitabine induces both radiographic and CA 19-9 tumor marker responses in patients with previously untreated advanced pancreatic cancer. *Journal of Clinical Oncology* **20**, 1182–1191.

Rothenberg, L. M., Moore, M. J., Cripps, M. C., Andersen, J. S., Portenoy, R. K., Burris, H. A. III *et al.* (1996). A phase II trial of gemcitabine in patients with 5-FU-refactory pancreas cancer. *Annals of Oncology* **7**, 347–353.

Ryan, D. P., Kulke, M. H., Fuchs, C. S., Grossbard, M. L., Grossman, S. R., Morgan, J. A. *et al.* (2002). A Phase II study of gemcitabine and docetaxel in patients with metastatic pancreatic carcinoma. *Cancer* **94**, 97–103.

Scheithauer, W., Schull, B., Ulrich-Pur, H., Schmid, K., Raderer, M., Haider, K. *et al.* (2003). Biweekly high-dose gemcitabine alone or in combination with capecitabine in patients with metastatic pancreatic adenocarcinoma: a randomized phase II trial. *Annals of Oncology* **14**, 97–104.

Stathopoulos, G. P., Mavroudis, D., Tsavaris, N., Kouroussis, C., Aravantinos, G., Agelaki, S. *et al.* (2001). Treatment of pancreatic cancer with a combination of docetaxel, gemcitabine and granulocyte colony-stimulating factor: a phase II study of the Greek Cooperative Group for Pancreatic Cancer. *Annals of Oncology* **12**, 101–103.

Stathopoulos, G. P., Rigatos, S. K., Dimopoulos, M. A., Giannakakis, T., Foutzilas, G., Kouroussis, C. *et al.* (2003). Treatment of pancreatic cancer with a combination of irinotecan (CPT-11) and gemcitabine: a multicenter phase II study by the Greek Cooperative Group for Pancreatic Cancer. *Annals of Oncology* **14**, 388–394.

Storniolo, A. M., Enas, N. H., Brown, C. A., Voi, M., Rothenberg, M. L. & Schilsky, R. (1999). An investigational new drug treatment program for patients with gemcitabine: results for over 3000 patients with pancreatic carcinoma. *Cancer* **85**, 1261–1268.

Tempero, M., Plunkett, W., Ruiz, V. H., Hainsworth, J., Hochster, H., Lenzi, R. *et al.* (2003). Randomized phase II comparison of dose-intense gemcitabine: thirty-minute infusion and fixed dose rate infusion in patients with pancreatic adenocarcinoma. *Journal of Clinical Oncology* **21**, 3402–3408.

Xiong, H. Q. & Abbruzzese, J. L. (2002). Epidermal growth factor receptor-targeted therapy for pancreatic cancer. *Seminars in Oncology* **29** (5 Suppl. 14), 31–37.

Chapter 11

Investigation and management of biliary tract cancer

Anne C. Armstrong and Juan W. Valle

Introduction

Biliary tract cancers include cancers of the gall bladder, cholangiocarcinomas and tumours of the ampulla of Vater. Cancers of the biliary tract are rare, accounting for around 1% of all reported tumours in the UK. With an annual incidence of 1.8 (males) and 2.8 (females) per 100,000, approximately 1200 cases are registered annually in England and Wales. The 1- and 5-year survivals for 1986–1990 (England and Wales) were 22% and 9%, respectively (Quinn *et al.* 2001). Gall bladder cancer is more common in women than men, with a peak incidence in the seventh decade of life, whereas cholangiocarcinomas are slightly more common in men and most frequently diagnosed in the fifth and sixth decades of life.

Cholangiocarcinomas are often described according to their location within the biliary tree. Perihilar (or Klatskin (Klatskin 1965)) tumours are the commonest, accounting for approximately two-thirds of tumours, with tumours distal to the origin of the common bile duct accounting for a further quarter and intrahepatic lesions the remainder (Nakeeb *et al.* 1996). Multifocal or diffuse involvement of the biliary tree is uncommon. Perihilar tumours were further classified by Bismuth *et al.* into four subtypes as tumours below the confluence of the right and left hepatic duct (type I), tumours reaching the confluence (type II), tumours extending beyond the confluence to either the right or left hepatic duct (type III), and tumours extending bilaterally to involve both ducts (type III) (Bismuth *et al.* 1992).

Risk factors

Disorders that produce chronic inflammation of the biliary tract appear to be associated with an increased risk of malignancy. For gall bladder tumours the epidemiology is similar to that of gallstones, though it remains unclear if this represents common risk factors or is cause and effect. Nevertheless, only 0.3–3% of patients with gallstones develop cancer of the gall bladder. Other risk factors include pancreatico-biliary duct junction anomalies, chronic typhoid infections and calcification of the gall bladder. Some chemicals, including methyldopa, isoniazid and chemicals used in the rubber industry have been implicated in carcinogenesis; no definitive proof is available (Zatonski *et al.* 1997).

Cholangiocarcinomas are more prevalent in Southeast Asia than other parts of the world, where the high incidence appears to be related to infection with the liver flukes *Clonorchis sinensis* and *Opisthorchis viverrini* (Kurathong *et al.* 1985; Schwartz, 1986). As with gall bladder tumours, other disorders that produce chronic inflammation of the biliary tract are associated with an increased risk of developing cholangiocarcinoma. In the West, the autoimmune disease, primary sclerosing cholangitis (PSC), is most often associated with the development of cholangiocarcinoma, with incidence rates ranging from 9–40% (Rosen *et al.* 1991; Cherqui *et al.* 1995; Van Laethem *et al.* 1995). Congenital cystic disease of the biliary tree is also associated with an increased risk of cholangiocarcinoma, presumably because of chronic inflammation within the biliary tract. The risk of cancer can be significantly reduced by early excision of the cysts (Becker *et al.* 1993).

Pathology

Gall bladder tumours can be categorised according to their growth pattern into infiltrative, nodular, papillary or combined forms; the commonest being infiltrative or combined nodular infiltrative forms. Infiltrative carcinomas may be difficult to distinguish from a chronically inflamed, benign gall bladder, whereas nodular carcinomas are more distinctive. Histologically, most gall bladder tumours are of epithelial cell origin (adenocarcinomas being the commonest subtype); more rarely, tumours may be of mesenchymal origin (Sumiyoshi *et al.* 1991).

Cholangiocarcinomas can be divided macroscopically into three subtypes: sclerosing, nodular and papillary (Weinbren & Mutum 1983). Sclerosing cholangiocarcinomas (seen as annular thickening of the bile duct) are the most frequent. Nodular tumours project into the lumen of the bile duct. When features of both subtypes are seen, the tumour is described as nodular-sclerosing. Papillary tumours are more friable, with less transmural involvement. They are more common in the distal bile duct and have a more favourable prognosis than the other two subtypes (Pitt *et al.* 1995). Most cholangiocarcinomas are mucin-secreting adenocarcinomas. The mucin or bile is useful to distinguish an intrahepatic cholangiocarcinoma from a hepatocellular carcinoma. A rare, clear cell variant of cholangiocarcinoma exists, which must be differentiated from renal clear-cell carcinoma with liver metastasis (Yamamoto *et al.* 1998).

Biliary tract cancers are staged according to the tumour-node-metastasis (TNM) system (AJCC, 1997). Staging varies for each type of biliary cancer. In general, in stage I tumour is limited to the mucosa or muscle layer. In stage II local invasion of tumour is seen, in stage III there are metastasis into regional lymph nodes with or without local invasion of tumour. In stage IV there is extensive tumour invasion of the liver or other local structures, non-regional lymph node involvement and distant metastases.

Clinical presentation

Most patients present with symptoms of biliary duct obstruction: jaundice, dark urine, pale stools and pruritus. Other common symptoms include abdominal pain, fever and weight-loss. The more friable papillary cholangiocarcinomas may detach and pass into and occlude the common bile duct causing intermittent jaundice. Peripheral or intra-hepatic cholangiocarcinomas and gall bladder tumours are often asymptomatic in early stages. Most patients present late, with advanced disease and with symptoms similar to that of hepatocellular carcinoma, including right upper quadrant, epigastric pain and weight loss. Jaundice is less common than distal or perihilar bile duct cancer, occurring in only 24% of patients (Chen 1999). Occasionally pancreatitis is the first manifestation of a periampullary tumour.

Investigations

Tumour markers

The most widely used serum tumour marker in biliary tract malignancies, in particular cholangiocarcinomas, is CA19-9. One study found elevated levels in over 80% of patients with cholangiocarcinoma; however, CA19-9 levels were also elevated in other tumour types (gastric, pancreatic and hepatocellular carcinomas) as well as (moderately elevated) in some benign pancreatic, liver and biliary conditions (Jalanko *et al.* 1984). This tumour marker has been studied as a means of screening patients with PSC who are at increased risk of developing the tumour. However, only 50% of patients developing the tumour had an elevated CA19-9, and the specificity of the marker in diagnosing the disease was again low (Hultcrantz *et al.* 1999). In addition, false-elevations of CA19-9 may be produced by cholangitis (Collazos *et al.* 1992). Serum carcino-embryonic antigen (CEA) levels are elevated in 40–60% of patients with cholangiocarcinoma (Jalanko *et al.* 1984; Nakeeb *et al.* 1996). In peripheral cholangiocarcinoma, unlike hepatocellular carcinoma, alpha-feto protein levels (AFP) are abnormal in less than 5% of patients (Nakeeb *et al.* 1996).

Radiology

Most patients are initially investigated with trans-abdominal ultrasound. Whereas small perihilar, extra-hepatic and periampullary tumours may not be directly visualised, there may be indirect signs of lesions such as ductal dilatation. Under optimal conditions ultrasound is able to detect up to 50% of gall bladder tumours (Bach *et al.* 1998) and up to 86% of cholangiocarcinomas (Hann *et al.* 1997). Computed tomography (CT) scans given further information about suspicious lesions, with intravenous bolus-enhanced spiral or helical CT scan able to provide information about the location of an obstructing tumour and the extent of tumour involvement (Tillich *et al.* 1998). Further useful investigations to assess potential resectability include angiography to determine arterial and portal venous vascular involvement and cholangiography to determine the location and extent of biliary disease. More recently, magnetic resonance cholangio-pancreatography (MRCP) and magnetic resonance angiography (MRA) have emerged as non-invasive replacements for cholangiography and angiography, respectively (Fulcher & Turner 2002). Tissue diagnosis of malignancy is often difficult with the yield depending on the modality used (cytological examination of bile: 30–40%; brush biopsy and cytology: 40–70%; percutaneous fine needle-aspirations/biopsy: 60%)(de Groen et al. 1999).

Surgical management of biliary tract cancer

Surgical resection is the only treatment modality that can potentially cure patients with biliary tract cancer. Stage 0 and I gall bladder cancers can be cured with laparoscopic cholecystectomy and are often found as an incidental finding on pathological examination. A 90–100% 3-year survival or stage II tumours (i.e. invasion through the muscle wall) is achieved by more extensive surgery (including resection of adjacent hepatic segments and regional lymph node clearance) (Bartlett 2000). This may require a re-resection for incidentally found tumours (Fong et al. 1998). Selected patients with locally advanced (Stage III/IV), node-negative tumors may also benefit from an extended resection (Bartlett 2000).

The appropriate surgery for cholangiocarcinomas depends on the site of the primary tumour. Intrahepatic tumours may be dealt with by hepatic resection alone; perihilar lesions may require resection of the extra-hepatic bile ducts, gall bladder, regional nodes, and formation of a draining hepatico-jejunostomy; while pancreatico-duodenectomy is indicated for distal tumours (Klempnauer et al. 1997; Madariaga et al. 1998; Reding et al. 1991).

Late presentation often precludes potentially curative surgery. However, other reasons may deem a patient inoperable: these are often elderly patients who may be medically unfit for an operation due to concurrent medical problems or ongoing liver failure and sepsis. Surgical therapy has an important role in the palliation of inoperable biliary tract disease, with biliary sepsis or liver failure often causing more life-threatening complications than metastatic disease. Endoscopically or percutaneously placed drainage and stents are able to relieve the symptoms caused by cholestasis. Metal stents have a larger diameter than plastic stents and tend to stay patent longer (Schima et al. 1997). Biliary enteric bypass can be an alternative to endobiliary stents, particularly when tumours are found to be unresectable at laparotomy.

Radiotherapy of biliary tract cancers
Adjuvant radiation therapy

Most patients who have undergone even potentially curative surgery still have a poor prognosis. Attempts have been made to improve the prognosis of these patients using adjuvant radiotherapy and several studies have confirmed the safety of both external beam and intraluminal brachytherapy in patients with biliary tract malignancies.

These tumours are, however, uncommon and the studies reported to date consist of small, non-randomised trials or retrospective case series using diverse regimens (including external beam irradiation, intra-operative radiotherapy, brachytherapy and intensity modulated radiotherapy), investigating differing endpoints and often treating a mixture of tumour types. It is difficult therefore to conclude that adjuvant radiation therapy has a significant impact on the disease.

One early retrospective study found an improved median survival of 63 months compared with 29 months for patients receiving post-operative radiation versus surgery alone for gall bladder tumours (Vaittinen 1970). Since this initial encouraging result, subsequent studies have produced mixed results; no added benefit of radiotherapy over surgery alone was seen in a cholangiocarcinoma study (Pitt *et al.* 1995). A similar study by the French Surgical Association compared survival of patients who had received surgery alone with those who received postoperative irradiation. No difference in overall survival was found, although there was a non-statistically significant trend for improved survival in favour of adjuvant radiation therapy (Reding *et al.* 1991). However, both in this and an earlier study, the addition of radiotherapy to palliative surgery appeared to extend survival (Cameron *et al.* 1990). Several other case series indicate that adjuvant radiotherapy in various modalities (Treadwell & Hardin, 1976; Bosset *et al.* 1989; Todoroki *et al.* 1991; Wolkov *et al.* 1992; Gonzalez Gonzalez *et al.* 1999; Urego *et al.* 1999; Mehta *et al.* 2001) can be given safely with varying degrees of benefit although without adequate control groups the evidence of efficacy is unsupported. Although the current evidence remains in favour of complete surgical resection as the cornerstone of treatment (Urego *et al.* 1999), confirmation of the benefit of adjuvant radiotherapy requires a prospective randomised study. Despite current 'optimal' therapy, only around one-quarter of patients are reaching 5-year survival (Koyama *et al.* 1993; Gonzalez Gonzalez *et al.* 1999; Urego *et al.* 1999).

Radiotherapy for advanced disease

Radiation therapy may also be given as a palliative measure in patients with locally advanced, inoperable disease. As with adjuvant therapy published clinical trials are generally small phase II trials and there is therefore no conclusive benefit of palliative radiotherapy either in terms of tumour response or improvements in quality of life. Furthermore, depending on the dose used and exposure to the normal tissues, radiotherapy can be associated with significant morbidity. Potential side effects include cholangitis, duodenitis and ulceration, hepatic artery stenosis, hepatic artery aneurysm, haemobilia and duodenal stenosis.

Few studies have investigated the palliative benefit of radiotherapy. Kopelson *et al.* (1977) reported good palliation with radiotherapy in terms of pruritus, pain or mass effect in four out of five patients with advanced gall bladder cancer with a radiation dose range from 38 to 50 Gy. In contrast, in another small study of patients with advanced biliary tract cancer only one of five patients achieved symptomatic benefit (Smoron 1977). A larger study of 41 patients with gall-bladder cancer looked at the benefit of radiotherapy following on from palliative surgery and found that patients treated with radiotherapy survived longer and with fewer symptoms than patients not receiving radiotherapy (Treadwell & Hardin 1976).

No benefit in terms of survival has been shown with palliative external beam radiotherapy. In one series, 6 of 22 patients with biliary tract cancer and residual disease post resection had no survival advantage over untreated patients, with all 22 patients dying within 11 months of diagnosis (Mittal *et al.* 1985). The radiation dose administered ranged from 12.5 to 59.4 Gy. Similar survival was seen in a later series of patients (Shiina *et al.* 1992) also treated with external beam radiotherapy, with a dose range of 26–78 Gy.

Intra-luminal brachytherapy (ILB), in which radioactive wires are inserted into the biliary tract by means of endoscopic or trans-hepatic stents or nasobiliary tubes, allow the administration of (high) doses of localised radiotherapy, reducing the risk of damage to surrounding tissues. In 1985 Karani *et al.* reported a survival advantage of 17 months against 8.5 months for untreated historical controls with the use of ILB (Karani *et al.* 1985). One disadvantage of ILB is that it may under-dose disease more than a centimetre distance from the radioactive wire. For this reason, particularly in the context of locally advanced disease, ILB is often given in combination with external beam radiotherapy (Buskirk *et al.* 1984; Flickinger *et al.* 1991; Fritz *et al.* 1994). A small comparative study found a median survival of 9 months when patients were treated with ILB alone as compared with 16 months with the addition of external beam radiotherapy (Johnson *et al.* 1985). In one study, 27 patients with biliary duct cancer were treated with ILB; 22 of these patients also received external beam radiotherapy. The median survival of the three patients receiving ILB alone was 3.6 months, compared with 14.3 months with combination radiotherapy (Meyers & Jones 1988). A recent study aimed to determine whether a dose–response existed for bile duct cancers treated with a combination of external beam radiotherapy and ILB. 18 patients were treated in three cohorts of one, two or three consecutive weeks of EBRT and ILB (total dose 52, 59 or 66 Gy). With increased dose of radiation there appeared to be a survival advantage with a median survival of 9, 12.2 and 20.3 months, though this failed to reach statistical significance. The treatment was well tolerated with one patient in the middle dose developing grade III toxicity (Lu *et al.* 2002).

Another approach that allows targeting of the radiation field to the tumour itself in an attempt to reduce the toxicity to normal tissues is intra-operative radiotherapy. Todorki *et al.* (1991) reported a series of 11 patients with stage IV gall bladder tumours and found a potential advantage of intra-operative radiation therapy at a dose of 30 Gy. The 3-year survival for the patients that received intra-operative radiotherapy was 10% against a 0% survival for patients those not treated with radiotherapy. It should be noted, however, that this latter group of patients did not receive radiotherapy because of the presence of liver or peritoneal metastases and were therefore likely to have a poorer prognosis than those patients with disease amenable to some sort of surgical resection. In another trial 20 patients with bile duct cancer were treated with intra-operative radiotherapy in addition to surgery. Nineteen of these patients had palliative resections only. The two-year survival of these 19 patients was 17% in comparison to 9% in a cohort of control patients. Patients included in the early part of the study received 27.5 Gy with this dose level being complicated by hepatic artery stenosis and aneurysms. Reducing the radiation dose to 20 Gy over a smaller field reduced the toxicity. It is not clear in this small group of patients whether this dose reduction also resulted in a reduction in efficacy (Iwasaki *et al.* 1988). In 1992 the Radiation Oncology Group (RTOG) reported a phase I/II study investigating the use of IORT for unresected, residual or locally recurrent biliary duct cancers (Wolkov *et al.* 1992). In eight patients treated there was one late grade 4 toxicity and minor complications were also common.

Chemo-radiotherapy

Systemic treatment with fluoropyrimidines has been successfully used in several tumours to sensitise tissues to the effects of radiation. A phase I study performed by the Eastern Oncology Group treated 9 patients with biliary tract malignancies and 16 patients with pancreatic cancer with escalating doses of 5-fluorouracil (5-FU) and combined with 59.4 Gy radiation fractionated over 6–7 weeks. The maximal tolerated dose of 5-FU was 250 mg/m^2, with oral mucositis as the dose-limiting toxicity rather than toxicities associated with radiation (Whittington *et al.* 1995). Other studies have demonstrated that chemoradiotherapy, using a variety of regimens, including hepatic arterial bromodeoxyuridine (Robertson *et al.* 1997) and mitomycin-C (MMC) (Minsky *et al.* 1991; Koyama *et al.* 1993), is, on the whole, well tolerated. One study treated patients with locally advanced pancreatic (19 patients), bile duct (7 patients) and gall bladder (1 patient) cancers with 40 Gy radiation and 350 mg/m^2 5-FU for 5 days. Eight patients developed grade III or IV toxicities, with toxicity greatest in elderly patients (older than 70 years) or those with a poor performance status (Hsue *et al.* 1996).

Chemotherapy

Fluoropyrimidine-based chemotherapy

5-Fluorouracil monotherapy

Given that 5-FU has been an integral drug in the treatment of most gastrointestinal malignancies, it is not surprising to find that most of the phase II studies performed to date are 5-FU-based (see Table 11.1). Two recent studies have shown very similar response rates (32–33%) and median survivals (6–7 months); one using a bolus 5-FU regimen (Choi *et al.* 2000), the other using 24-hour infusional 5-FU (Chen *et al.* 1998), both modulated by leucovorin. In one arm of the randomised EORTC 40955 phase II study, the median survival was comparable although the response rate was only 7% with 44% of patients achieving stable disease (Mitry *et al.* 2002).

Table 11.1 5-Fluorouracil-based phase II studies

Chemotherapy	n	CC	GB	RR (%)	SD (%)	MS (mo)	Study
5-FU	29			7	44	5.3	Mitry et al. 2002
5-FU/FA	19	13	6	33	39	7	Chen et al. 1998
5-FU/FA	28			32		6	Choi et al. 2000
5-FU + MMC + doxorubicin	17			31	41	—	Harvey et al. 1984
5-FU + MMC + doxorubicin (modified)	42			7			Takada et al. 1998
5-FU/FA + MMC	25	22	3	26	42	6	Chen et al. 2001
5-FU/FA + MMC	20			25	30	10	Raderer et al. 1999
5-FU + MMC (IHA)	11			64*		12+	Smith et al. 1984
5-FU/FA + carboplatin	14			21*	29	5	Sanz-Altamira et al. 1998
5-FU + cisplatin	25			24	—	—	Ducreux et al. 1998
5-FU/FA + cisplatin	29			19*	37	7.8	Mitry et al. 2002
5-FU/FA + cisplatin	29			34*	38	28	Taieb et al. 2002
5-FU + cisplatin + epirubicin	25	—	—	40	—	—	Ellis et al. 1995
5-FU + cisplatin + epirubicin	15	9	6	33*	33	9.5	Di Lauro et al. 1997
5-FU + cisplatin + epirubicin	24	0	24	29	13	6.4	Okada et al. 1997
5-FU + IFN	35	25	10	34		12	Patt et al. 1996
5-FU + IFN + cisplatin + doxorubicin	22	22	0	9		18	Patt et al. 2001
5-FU + IFN + cisplatin + doxorubicin	19	0	19	35		11	Patt et al. 2001
5-FU + MTX + epirubicin	22	11	6	0			Kajanti & Pyrhonen, 1994
5-FU/FA + hydroxyurea	30	0	30	30	27	8	Gebbia et al. 1996

n, Total number of patients in the study; where specified, the number of patients with cholangiocarcinomas (CC) or gall bladder tumours (GB) is also given. RR, response rate; SD, stable disease; MS, median survival. *Includes complete responses.

5-Fluorouracil and mitomycin-C combinations

To optimise efficacy, various 5-FU combination studies have been reported. Harvey et al. (1984) published a phase II trial using a combination of 5-FU 600 mg/m^2 on days 1 and 8, doxorubicin 30 mg/m^2 and MMC 10 mg/m^2 (FAM) on day 1 in 17 patients with advanced biliary carcinoma. Four of 14 patients (31%) with measurable disease achieved a partial response. More recently, Raderer et al. investigated the use of bolus 5-FU (400 mg/m^2), leucovorin (200 mg/m^2) on days 1-4 and MMC (8 mg/m^2) on day 1 (Raderer et al. 1999) in 20 patients with biliary tract malignancies. The overall response rate in this study was 25% with a 9.5-month median survival. MMC (10 mg/m^2) has also been given in combination with 24-hour infusional 5-FU (Chen et al. 2001) with a response rate of 26% in 25 patients with biliary tract cancers. Four patients died on study, leading the authors to conclude that the regimen causes increased toxicity without improving the response rate compared with 5-FU alone. Increasing dose intensity by the administration of intra-hepatic arterial 5-FU and MMC may increase both response rate and survival, although this has not been compared with peripheral administration in a prospective randomised study (Smith *et al.* 1984).

5-Fluorouracil and platinum combinations

A 25-patient study with locally advanced or metastatic biliary tract cancers using a 5-day continuous infusion of 5-FU $1g/m^2$/day with cisplatin 100 mg/m^2 on day 2 achieved six partial remissions (response rate 24%) (Ducreux *et al.* 1998). The same group recently reported the results of adding leucovorin to a modified 5-FU/cisplatin combination. Twenty-nine patients were treated with leucovorin 200 mg/m^2, 5-FU 400 mg/m^2 bolus followed by a 22-hour continuous infusion of 600 mg/m^2 for two days with cisplatin at 50 mg/m^2 on day 2 (Taieb *et al.* 2002). Responses were seen in 10 patients (34%) with one complete and nine partial responses. The regimen was reasonably well tolerated with one grade 4 thrombocytopaenia, although grade 3 toxicities occurred in 41% of patients. On behalf of the EORTC, the results of a randomised phase II study were recently presented (Mitry *et al.* 2002). Patients ($n = $ 29 in each arm) with biliary tract cancer were randomised to receiving 5-FU $3g/m^2$ over 24 hours weekly for six weeks or 5-FU (2.6 g/m^2 over 24 hours) in combination with folinic acid (500 mg/m^2) and cisplatin 50 mg/m^2. Although the response rate and median survivals in the 5-FU alone arm versus the combination arm were 7% versus 19% and 5.3 versus 7.8 months respectively, the small patient numbers do not allow formal statistical comparison. In an attempt to minimise renal toxicity, Sanz-Altamira *et al.* used carboplatin 300 mg/m^2 on day 1 with 5-FU 400 mg/m^2 with leucovorin 25 mg/m^2 on days 1–4 of a 28-day cycle. Three responses (21.4%, one complete and two partial) were seen among the 14 patients treated (Sanz-Altamira *et al.* 1998).

Three studies have looked at adding epirubicin to the cisplatin-5-FU combination. Epirubicin 50 mg/m^2 with cisplatin (60 mg/m^2) on day 1 and continuous infusional 5-FU (200 mg/m^2/d, days 1–21) (ECF, 21-day regimen) resulted in a 40% response rate (with a 10-month duration of response) among 25 patients with biliary tumours. A further 25% attained disease stabilisation with an overall median survival of 11 months and manageable toxicity (Ellis *et al.* 1995). In a smaller study, 15 patients received cisplatin 25 mg/m^2, epirubicin 20 mg/m^2 and 5-FU 500 mg/m^2, each on days 1–3, every 4 weeks. 5 responses were seen (1 complete and 4 partial), with a median time to progression of 4 months and overall survival of 9.5 months (Di Lauro *et al.* 1997). The third study treated only patients with gall bladder cancer ($n = 24$) with cisplatin 80 mg/m^2 and epirubicin 50 mg/m^2 on day 1, and continuous 5-FU infusion 500 mg/m^2/d on days 1–5. The RR was 29% and overall survival 6.4 months (Okada *et al.* 1997).

5-Fluorouracil with interferon modulation

Patt *et al.* have published two studies modulating 5-FU with systemic recombinant interferon (rIFN) α-2b. 35 patients with unresectable cancer of the biliary tree were treated with infusional 5-FU (750 mg/m^2/day) on days 1–5 with rIFN (5 MU/m^2) on days 1, 3 and 5, every 2 weeks. Eleven patients (34%) had a partial response (Patt *et al.* 1996) with a median survival of 12 months. Based on these results, the regimen was intensified by the addition of cisplatin 80 mg/m^2 and doxorubicin 40 mg/m^2 to 5-FU (500 mg/m^2, continuous infusion, days 1–3) and rIFN (5 MU/m^2, daily for 4 days). The regimen was more active for gall bladder tumours than cholangiocarcinomas, with a response rate of 35% compared with 9%; however, it was also associated with a marked increase in toxicity (Patt *et al.* 2001).

Other 5-fluorouracil combinations

5-FU, modulated with leucovorin and given in combination with oral hydroxyurea had a response rate of 30% in a study of 30 patients with advanced gall bladder tumours (Gebbia *et al.* 1996). Toxicity of the treatment was mild, with gastrointestinal toxicities most common. 5-FU and epirubicin have also been given in combination with methotrexate (MTX) (Kajanti & Pyrhonen 1994). Patients received 20 mg/m^2 of epirubicin, 150 mg/m^2 MTX and 600 mg/m^2 5-FU every week for 3 weeks with 2–3 weeks rest between cycles. No tumour responses were seen with this regimen.

Oral fluoropyrimidines

In a prospective randomised phase II study, the Eastern Cooperative Oncology Group compared the efficacy oral 5-FU monotherapy with oral 5-FU plus intravenous streptozotocin or lomustine (methyl-CCNU) in patients with advanced biliary cancer. In total, 53 patients with advanced gall bladder cancer and 34 patients with advanced bile duct cancer were included. Efficacy was limited with an overall response rate of less than 10%, with no significant difference between the treatment arms either in response rates or overall survival (Falkson *et al.* 1984).

A more recent study investigated the use of uracil/tegafur (UFT) 300 mg/m^2/day modulated with 90 mg/day leucovorin for 28 days, repeated every 35 days. No complete or partial responses were seen among 13 patients with advanced, measurable, biliary tract cancer, although 31% attained stable disease (Mani *et al.* 1999). More encouragingly, the oral pro-drug capecitabine induced tumour responses in 50% of gall bladder cancer patients (including two complete responses) although only 6% of cholangiocarcinomas responded in a study by Lozano *et al.* (2000). An ongoing study adding cisplatin to capecitabine has, thus far, attained an overall response rate of 24%, with a median survival of more than 8 months (Kim *et al.* 2002) (see Table 11.2). Clearly, an oral fluoropyrimidine would result in improved patient convenience although the benefits of any such regimen would need to be validated in a prospective randomised trial.

Table 11.2 Oral fluoropyrimidine phase II studies

Chemotherapy	n	CC	GB	RR (%)	SD (%)	MS (mo)	Study
5-FU	30		CC 8	GB 11			Falkson *et al.* 1984
5-FU + STZ	26		0	12			Falkson *et al.* 1984
5-FU + meCCNU	31		17	5			Falkson *et al.* 1984
UFT + FA	13			0	31	7	Mani *et al.* 1999
Capecitabine	26	18	8	6 50*			Lozano *et al.* 2000
Capecitabine + cisplatin	21+	11	10	24	18	8+	Kim *et al.* 2002

n, Total number of patients in the study; where specified, the number of patients with cholangiocarcinomas (CC) or gall bladder tumours (GB) is also given. RR, response rate; SD, stable disease; MS, median survival. *Includes complete responses.

Gemcitabine-based regimens

Given the increasing use of gemcitabine for pancreatic cancer, a number of investigators have looked at phase II studies of single-agent gemcitabine for biliary tract cancers (Table 11.3). In the first to be published, 11 patients with biliary tract cancer were treated with gemcitabine at 1000 mg/m^2/week for seven weeks and then weekly for three out of four weeks. All patients received at least eight doses of gemcitabine but no objective tumour responses were seen (Mezger *et al.* 1997). However, recent studies have been more promising, with several small studies demonstrating radiological response rates of 22–45% (Verderame *et al.* 2000; Arroyo *et al.* 2001; Gallardo *et al.* 2001; Gebbia *et al.* 2001; Kubicka *et al.* 2001; Duck *et al.* 2002). Moreover, some studies appeared to demonstrate a 'clinical benefit' from chemotherapy with a relief of tumour symptoms, improved Karnofsky performance score (KP) or weight gain (Gallardo *et al.* 2002; Kubicka *et al.* 2001; Verderame *et al.* 2000). Increasing the dose of gemcitabine to 1200 mg/m^2/week for 3 out of 4 weeks (Raderer *et al.* 1999) or to 2200 mg/m^2 every 14 days (Penz *et al.* 2001), although well tolerated, does not obviously appear to increase efficacy. Neither does a prolonged, fixed-rate infusion of 10 mg/m^2/min, which did, however, result in enhanced (haematological) toxicity (Dragovich *et al.* 2000).

Gemcitabine is increasingly being studied in combination with other drugs (Table 11.4). The response rate to a combination of gemcitabine and irinotecan is modest and is associated with significant haematological toxicity. There were two deaths (from progressive disease and non-neutropaenic pneumonia) in a cohort of 14 patients (Jani *et al.* 2002). An ongoing study of docetaxel in combination with gemcitabine has produced a response rate of 9% with 55% attaining disease stabilisation (Kuhn *et al.* 2001). An initial study of gemcitabine with capecitabine has produced a response rate of 29% although only 5 patients with biliary tract cancer were included among 25 patients with gastrointestinal malignancies (Campos *et al.* 2001).

146 Anne C. Armstrong and Juan W. Valle

Table 11.3 Single-agent gemcitabine phase II studies

Chemotherapy	n	CC	GB	RR (%)	SD (%)	MS (mo)	Study
Gemcitabine standard	11	8	3	0	55	-	Mezger et al. 1997
Gemcitabine standard	11	11	0	45	9	20	Duck et al. 2002
Gemcitabine standard	26	0	26	36	24	6.9	Gallardo et al. 2001
Gemcitabine standard	42	7	34	36*	28	6.5	Arroyo et al. 2001
Gemcitabine standard	23	23	0	30	—	—	Kubicka et al. 2001
Gemcitabine standard	18	6	12	22	28	8	Gebbia et al. 2001
Gemcitabine standard	4			25	75	—	Verderame et al. 2000
Gemcitabine 1200 mg/m^2 D1,8,15 q28d	19			16	21	6.5	Raderer et al. 1999
Gemcitabine 1500 (rate: 10mg/m^2/min)	13	5	8	8	50	—	Dragovich et al. 2000
Gemcitabine 2200 mg/m^2 q14d	32			22	44	11.5	Penz et al. 2001
IHA-Gemcitabine 1200 mg/m^2 q28d	8			25*	38	—	Weissmann & Ludwig, 1999

Gemcitabine standard = 1000 mg/m^2 D1,8,15 q28d +/– rest week on first month.
n, Total number of patients in the study; where specified, the number of patients with cholangiocarcinomas (CC) or gall bladder tumours (GB) is also given. RR, response rate; SD, stable disease; MS, median survival. *Includes complete responses.

Table 11.4 Gemcitabine combination phase II studies

Chemotherapy	n	CC	GB	RR (%)	SD (%)	MS (mo)	Study
Gemcitabine + irinotecan D1,8,15	14+	5	9	14	43	—	Jani et al. 2002
Gemcitabine + docetaxel D1,8,15	43	17	26	9	55	11	Kuhn et al. 2001
Gemcitabine + capecitabine D1-14	4+	3	1	—	—	—	Campos et al. 2001
Gemcitabine + cisplatin D1	30	0	30	53*	41	—	Doval et al. 2001
Gemcitabine + cisplatin D1,8,15	11	5	6	50*	40	11.3	Carraro et al. 2001

N, Total number of patients in the study; where specified, the number of patients with cholangiocarcinomas (CC) or gall bladder tumours (GB) is also given. RR, response rate; SD, stable disease; MS; median survival. *Includes complete responses.

The most promising combination, based on phase II studies, may be the combination of gemcitabine with cisplatin. Carraro *et al.*, treated 11 patients with biliary tract cancer with gemcitabine 1000 mg/m^2 and cisplatin 30 mg/m^2 for 3 out of every 4 weeks (Carraro *et al.* 2001). The response rate was 50%, with two complete responses; however, there were two deaths (cerebral ischaemia and unknown cause) during treatment in this small group. A second study administered a 21-day cycle of gemcitabine 1000 mg/m^2 on days 1 and 8, with cisplatin at 70 mg/m^2 on day 1 only to 30 patients with gall bladder cancers (Doval *et al.* 2001). Again this combination of drugs looks promising, with a response rate of 53% including six complete responses and a further 41% of patients with stable disease. No median survival has been reported, and the toxicity was described as 'moderate'.

Other agents

In 1976 one of the earliest studies with mitomycin-C (MMC) reported a promising response rate of 47% in patients with biliary cancer (Crooke & Bradner 1976). Unfortunately, these response rates have not been duplicated since and in a subsequent European Organisation for Research and Treatment of Cancer (EORTC) study only 3 of 30 patients with unresectable biliary cancer treated with 6-weekly MMC 15 mg/m^2 had partial remissions leading the authors to conclude that single agent MMC had no significant activity in this patient group (Taal *et al.* 1993). Activity of MMC may be improved by selective intra-arterial administration (Makela & Kairaluoma 1993).

Cisplatin monotherapy has been largely shown to be ineffective with two phase II trials, reporting a partial response rate in 0 out of 9 patients (Ravry *et al.* 1986) and 1 out of 13 patients (Okada *et al.* 1994) treated. Interestingly, a small study using a carboplatin-coated stent achieved a response in three out of five patients with stable disease in the other two (Mezawa *et al.* 2000) although the additional benefits over adequate stenting alone have yet to be shown.

Newer agents such as the taxanes appear to have limited activity: paclitaxel at a dose of 170–200 mg/m^2 every 21 days produced no responses in 15 patients with unresectable bile duct and gall-bladder cancer (Jones *et al.* 1996). Docetaxel, at a dose of 100 mg/m^2 every 21 days, was also shown to be ineffective in a cohort of 17 patients with unresectable cholangiocarcinoma (Pazdur *et al.* 1999). Furthermore, one patient died of septic shock shortly after starting the study. In contrast, another group using an identical regimen of docetaxel achieved an overall response rate of 20% (including complete responses) with no toxic deaths in a study of 25 patients (Papakostas *et al.* 2001).

Small studies have investigated the use of liposomal doxorubicin (Miller *et al.* 2002), irinotecan (Fishkin *et al.* 2001), raltitrexed (Francois *et al.* 2001), DX8951f (exatecan mesylate) (Abou-Alfa *et al.* 2002) and etoposide (Ekstrom *et al.* 1998), but all of these agents appear to be inactive in biliary tract cancer, and, in the case of irinotecan, associated with significant toxicity (see Table 11.5).

Table 11.5 Single-agent (non-fluoropyrimidine, non-gemcitabine) phase II studies.

Chemotherapy	n	CC	GB	RR (%)	SD (%)	MS (mo)	Study
MMC				47			Crooke & Bradner 1976
MMC	34			10			Taal *et al.* 1993
IA-MMC	25	0	25	44		13	Makela & Kairaluoma 1993
Cisplatin				0			Ravry *et al.* 1986
Cisplatin	13			8			Okada *et al.* 1994
Carboplatin-coated stent	5			60	40		Mezawa *et al.* 2000
Paclitaxel	15	11	4	0			Jones *et al.* 1996
Docetaxel	17	17	0	0	6	-	Pazdur *et al.* 1999
Docetaxel	25			20*	24	8	Papakostas *et al.* 2001
Liposomal doxorubicin	8	8	0	0			Miller *et al.* 2002
Irinotecan	21	0	21	11		6	Fishkin *et al.* 2001
DX8951f (exatecan)	42	25	17	5	40	10	Abou-Alfa *et al.* 2002
Raltitrexed	9			5	24	-	Francois *et al.* 2001

n, Total number of patients in the study; where specified, the number of patients with cholangiocarcinomas (CC) or gall bladder tumours (GB) is also given. RR, response rate, SD, stable disease; MS, median survival. *Includes complete responses.

Randomised studies

Given the many small phase II studies previously discussed, it is disappointing to find only two prospectively randomised studies. A Swedish study enrolled a mixture of 53 pancreatic and 37 biliary tract cancer patients (total 93 patients). Patients were randomised to receive either best supportive care (BSC) or chemotherapy with the FELv regimen (5-FU 500 mg/m^2, etoposide 120 mg/m^2 and leucovorin 60 mg/m^2 on days 1–3 of a 21-day regimen). Etoposide was omitted in the elderly and for patients with poor performance score. Forty-three patients were allocated BSC (24 pancreas, 19 biliary) and 27 to chemotherapy (29 pancreas, 18 biliary). Delayed chemotherapy was allowed for patients allocated BSC, and was given to 8 of the 43 patients. Although the response rate was not an endpoint for the study, 39 patients in the chemotherapy arm were assessable; the response rate was low (8%) with stable disease 38% and progressive disease 54%. Forty-one per cent of patients receiving the FELv regimen experienced grade 3–4 toxicity, with the proportion highest in patients older than 60 years. Despite this, patients who received chemotherapy had a delayed time to disease progression (4 versus 1.5 months) and significantly better quality of life scores (QLQ-C30). There was an improved survival when considering all patients (6 versus 2.5 months for pancreatic cancer and biliary cancers) which, while reaching the level of significance for pancreatic cancer patients ($p = 0.05$), was not so for biliary cancer ($p = 0.1$) (Glimelius *et al.* 1996).

A Japanese study randomised 83 patients with pancreatic ($n = 52$) and biliary carcinoma ($n = 31$) to palliative surgery alone or palliative surgery followed by a modified FAM regimen (5-FU, doxorubicin and MMC doses: 200 mg/m^2, 15 mg/m^2 and 5 mg/m^2, respectively, all given weekly for four weeks followed by a rest week, for 2 cycles). Median survivals for patients allocated FAM versus palliative surgery alone were 5.2 versus 2.4 months for gall bladder carcinomas and 4.0 versus 7.6 months for biliary tract carcinomas. Two of ten patients (20%) with gall bladder carcinoma responded to treatment with a further patient (10%) having stable disease. All patients with biliary tract cancers progressed on chemotherapy. However, with only a total of 18 patients with gall bladder carcinoma and 13 patients with biliary tract cancers this study is underpowered to make any conclusions about the efficacy of chemotherapy (Takada *et al.* 1998).

There is increasing evidence that biliary tract cancers, and maybe gall bladder cancer in particular, may be chemo-sensitive. Treatment looks most promising for fluoropyrimidines and gemcitabine-based regimens, although the lack of adequately powered, homogeneous, prospective randomised trials makes any conclusion of the optimal chemotherapy regimen hard to reach. Clearly, further, well-designed, randomised studies looking at the relative merits of selected chemotherapy drugs and regimens are warranted.

Photodynamic therapy

Another promising approach that may relieve biliary obstruction is the use of photodynamic therapy (PDT): a modality of treatment being increasingly used for many malignancies including oesophageal cancer, non-small cell lung cancer, papillary bladder cancer and cervical cancer. The principle behind this is that patients, pre-treated with a photosensitiser, can have a laser fibre inserted endoscopically or percutaneously into the biliary tract, through which laser therapy is given.

A study looking at the efficacy of PDT (using haematoporphyrin) in non-operable ampullary tumours achieved remissions in 3 of 10 treated patients. More importantly, the modality of treatment was shown to be safe, feasible and could be administered repeatedly (Abulafi *et al.* 1995). Pahernik *et al.* (1998) demonstrated that the sensitiser Photofrin reached peak concentrations in biliary malignancies during the first two days. Subsequent studies by the same German group have shown that cholestasis may be improved in some patients and treatment with PDT and biliary stenting may result in a survival advantage (with a 74% 6-month survival) although the added benefit over stenting alone needs to be confirmed in a prospective, randomised study (Berr *et al.* 2000a,b). Another group who treated eight patients with bile duct cancers with PDT in addition to standard biliary stenting demonstrated potential clinical efficacy of this therapy. A reduction in biliary duct stenosis was seen in all patients four weeks after PDT, with a consequent reduction in serum bilirubin (Zoepf *et al.* 2001a). Again the treatment was well tolerated, with two patients developing infectious complications. The technique is still undergoing adaptations of equipment (Rumalla *et al.* 2001) and photosensitiser (Zoepf *et al.* 2001b). These results have generated wide interest and collaboration between investigators to evaluate efficacy and feasibility on a greater scale, with the ultimate aim of a multi-centre randomised study, is currently underway.

Conclusions

Biliary tract cancers are rare malignancies that are often difficult to diagnose, and most patients present late with advanced, unresectable disease. Surgery offers the only potential for long-term cure but often requires technically difficult or extensive procedures, which may be associated with significant co-morbidity. Advances in imaging and surgical techniques over the past two decades have improved the outlook for some patients presenting with these tumours but the majority of cases still remain unresectable. Most patients succumb to tumour spread in the biliary tree, refractory cholestasis, and sepsis or liver failure. The optimal palliative care for these patients has not been adequately defined. Surgical drainage procedures to maintain biliary patency to relieve jaundice and reduce the risk of sepsis remain the mainstay of treatment for these patients. Many chemoradiotherapeutic regimes have been investigated in clinical trials, with some clinical or symptomatic responses. Because of the rarity of these tumours resulting in few patient numbers being treated across a relatively large number of institutions most of the trials have been small, non-randomised phase II trials (with heterogeneity of tumour types), and it is therefore difficult to conclude that any of the therapies tried have a significant effect on the natural course of the disease. Many questions remain over the role of the various modalities of treatment (PDT, radiotherapy and chemotherapy) at the various stages of disease (adjuvant, neo-adjuvant and advanced settings). For each of these settings, appropriate end-points must be defined (e.g. survival rather than response rate in advanced disease). Patients should, therefore, be encouraged to participate in well-designed, large (national and international collaborative) multicentre phase III trials to define the standard of care for these malignancies.

References

Abou-Alfa, G. K., O'Reilly, E. M., Rowinsky, E. K., Patt, Y., Schwartz, G. K., Sharma, S., Siegel, E., Eckhardt, S. G., Becerra, C., Jakubowitz, J., Duggal, A., Lubicz, S. & De Jager, R. (2002). Final results of a phase II study of DX-8951f (DX, exatecan mesylate) in biliary tree cancers. *Proceedings of the American Society of Clinical Oncology* **21**, 141a (abstract 561).

Abulafi, A. M., Allardice, J. T., Williams, N. S., van Someren, N., Swain, C. P. & Ainley, C. (1995). Photodynamic therapy for malignant tumours of the ampulla of Vater. *Gut*, **36**, 853–856.

AJCC (1997). Gallbladder and extrahepatic bile ducts. In *American Joint Committee on Cancer: AJCC Cancer Staging Manual.*, Fleming, I.D., Cooper, J.S. & Henson, D.E. (eds) pp. 103–113. Lippincott-Raven Publishers: Philadelphia, PA.

Arroyo, G., Gallardo, J., Rubio, B., Orlandi, L., Yanez, M., Gamargo, C., Ahumada, M., Zarba, J., Berlingeri, G. & Kowalyszyn, R. (2001). Gemcitabine (Gem) in advanced biliary tract cancer (ABTC). Experience from Chile and Argentina in phase II trials. *Proceedings of the American Society of Clinical Oncology* **20**, 157a (abstract 626).

Bach, A. M., Loring, L. A., Hann, L. E., Illescas, F. F., Fong, Y. & Blumgart, L. H. (1998). Gallbladder cancer: can ultrasonography evaluate extent of disease? *Journal of Ultrasound Medicine* **17**, 303–309.

Bartlett, D. L. (2000). Gallbladder cancer. *Seminars in Surgical Oncology* **19**, 145–155.

Becker, C. D., Glattli, A., Maibach, R. & Baer, H. U. (1993). Percutaneous palliation of malignant obstructive jaundice with the Wallstent endoprosthesis: follow-up and reintervention in patients with hilar and non-hilar obstruction. *Journal of Vascular Interventional Radiology* **4**, 597–604.

Berr, F., Tannapfel, A., Lamesch, P., Pahernik, S. A., Wiedmann, M., Halm, U., Goetz, A. E., Mossner, J. & Hauss, J. (2000a). Neoadjuvant photodynamic therapy before curative resection of proximal bile duct carcinoma. *Journal of Hepatology* **32**, 352–357.

Berr, F., Wiedmann, M., Tannapfel, A., Halm, U., Kohlhaw, K. R., Schmidt, F., Wittekind, C., Hauss, J. & Mossner, J. (2000b). Photodynamic therapy for advanced bile duct cancer: evidence for improved palliation and extended survival. *Hepatology* **31**, 291–298.

Bismuth, H., Nakache, R. & Diamond, T. (1992). Management strategies in resection for hilar cholangiocarcinoma. *Annals of Surgery* **215**, 31–38.

Bosset, J. F., Mantion, G., Gillet, M., Pelissier, E., Boulenger, M., Maingon, P., Corbion, O. & Schraub, S. (1989). Primary carcinoma of the gallbladder. Adjuvant postoperative external irradiation. *Cancer* **64**, 1843–1847.

Buskirk, S. J., Gunderson, L. L., Adson, M. A., Martinez, A., May, G. R., McIlrath, D. C., Nagorney, D. M., Edmundson, G. K., Bender, C. E. & Martin, J. K. Jr (1984). Analysis of failure following curative irradiation of gallbladder and extrahepatic bile duct carcinoma. *International Journal of Radiation Oncology, Biology, Physics* **10**, 2013–2023.

Cameron, J. L., Pitt, H. A., Zinner, M. J., Kaufman, S. L. & Coleman, J. (1990). Management of proximal cholangiocarcinomas by surgical resection and radiotherapy. *American Journal of Surgery* **159**, 91–97; discussion 97–98.

Campos, L. T., Alvarez, R., Sanford, D., Miro-Quesada, M., Holoye, P. & Manner, C. (2001). Gemcitabine (Gem) and capecitabine (CPC) in advanced pancreatic cancer (APC) and solid tumours. A single centre experience. *Proceedings of the American Society of Clinical Oncology* **20**, 141b (abstract 2315).

Carraro, S., Servienti, P. J., Bruno, M. F., Castillo Odena, M. D., Roca, E., Jovtis, S., Felci, N. & Araujo, C. (2001). Gemcitabine and cisplatin in locally advanced or metastatic gallbladder and bile duct adenocarcinomas. *Proceedings of the American Society of Clinical Oncology* **20**, 146b (abstract 2333).

Chen, J. S., Jan, Y. Y., Lin, Y. C., Wang, H. M., Chang, W. C. & Liau, C. T. (1998). Weekly 24 hour infusion of high-dose 5-fluorouracil and leucovorin in patients with biliary tract carcinomas. *Anticancer Drugs* **9**, 393–397.

Chen, J. S., Lin, Y. C., Jan, Y. Y. & Liau, C. T. (2001). Mitomycin C with weekly 24-h infusion of high-dose 5-fluorouracil and leucovorin in patients with biliary tract and periampullar carcinomas. *Anticancer Drugs* **12**, 339–343.

Chen, M. F. (1999). Peripheral cholangiocarcinoma (cholangiocellular carcinoma): clinical features, diagnosis and treatment. *Journal of Gastroenterology and Hepatology* **14**, 1144–1149.

Cherqui, D., Tantawi, B., Alon, R., Piedbois, P., Rahmouni, A., Dhumeaux, D., Julien, M. & Fagniez, P. L. (1995). Intrahepatic cholangiocarcinoma. Results of aggressive surgical management. *Archives of Surgery* **130**, 1073–1078.

Choi, C. W., Choi, I. K., Seo, J. H., Kim, B. S., Kim, J. S., Kim, C. D., Um, S. H. & Kim, Y. H. (2000). Effects of 5-fluorouracil and leucovorin in the treatment of pancreatic-biliary tract adenocarcinomas. *American Journal of Clinical Oncology* **23**, 425–428.

Collazos, J., Genolla, J. & Ruibal, A. (1992). CA19-9 in non-neoplastic liver diseases. A clinical and laboratory study. *Clinica Chimica Acta* **210**, 145–151.

Crooke, S. T. & Bradner, W. T. (1976). Mitomycin C: a review. *Cancer Treatment Reviews* **3**, 121–139.

de Groen, P. C., Gores, G. J., LaRusso, N. F., Gunderson, L. L. & Nagorney, D. M. (1999). Biliary tract cancers. *New England Journal of Medicine* **341**, 1368–1378.

Di Lauro, L., Carpano, S., Capomolla, E., Conti, F., Rinaldi, M., Lopez, M. & Vici, P. (1997). Cisplatin, epirubicin and fluorouracil (PEF) for advanced biliary tract carcinoma. *Proceedings of the American Society of Clinical Oncology* **16**, 287a (abstract 1021).

Doval, D. C., Sekhon, J. S., Fuloria, J., Gupta, S. K., Vaid, A. K., Gupta, S. & Shukla, V. K. (2001). Gemcitabine and cisplatin in chemotherapy naive, unresectable gallbladder cancer: a large multicentre, phase II study. *Proceedings of the American Society of Clinical Oncology* **20**, 156a (abstract 622).

Dragovich, T., Ramanthan, R. K., Remick, S., Dyky, M. A., Wade-Oliver, K. T., Jacobs, S., Mani, S. & Kindler, H. L. (2000). Phase II trial of a weekly 150-minute gemcitabine infusion in patients with biliary tree carcinomas. *Proceedings of the American Society of Clinical Oncology* **19**, 296a (abstract).

Duck, L., Humblet, Y., Gigot, J.-F., Lonneux, M., Baurain, J. F. & Machiels, J.-P. (2002). Gemcitabine in advanced cholangiocarcinoma: a single-centre retrospective study. *Proceedings of the American Society of Clinical Oncology* **21**, 125b (abstract 2314).

Ducreux, M., Rougier, P., Fandi, A., Clavero-Fabri, M. C., Villing, A. L., Fassone, F., Fandi, L., Zarba, J. & Armand, J. P. (1998). Effective treatment of advanced biliary tract carcinoma using 5-fluorouracil continuous infusion with cisplatin. *Annals of Oncology* **9**, 653–656.

Ekstrom, K., Hoffman, K., Linne, T., Eriksson, B. & Glimelius, B. (1998). Single-dose etoposide in advanced pancreatic and biliary cancer, a phase II study. *Oncology Reports* **5**, 931–934.

Ellis, P. A., Norman, A., Hill, A., O'Brien, M. E., Nicolson, M., Hickish, T. & Cunningham, D. (1995). Epirubicin, cisplatin and infusional 5-fluorouracil (5-FU) (ECF) in hepatobiliary tumours. *European Journal of Cancer* **31A**, 1594–1598.

Falkson, G., MacIntyre, J. M. & Moertel, C. G. (1984). Eastern Cooperative Oncology Group experience with chemotherapy for inoperable gallbladder and bile duct cancer. *Cancer* **54**, 965–969.

Fishkin, P., Alberts, S., Mahoney, M., Sargent, D., Goldberg, R., Burgart, L., Cera, P., Morton, R., Johnson, P. & Nair, S. (2001). Irinotecan (CPT-11) in patients with advanced gallbladder carcinoma: a North Central Cancer Treatment Group (NCCTG) phase II study. *Proceedings of the American Society of Clinical Oncology* **20**, 155a (abstract 618).

Flickinger, J. C., Epstein, A. H., Iwatsuki, S., Carr, B. I. & Starzl, T. E. (1991). Radiation therapy for primary carcinoma of the extrahepatic biliary system. An analysis of 63 cases. *Cancer* **68**, 289–294.

Fong, Y., Heffernan, N. & Blumgart, L. H. (1998). Gallbladder carcinoma discovered during laparoscopic cholecystectomy: aggressive reresection is beneficial. *Cancer* **83**, 423–427.

Francois, E., Hebbar, M., Bennouna, D., Mayeur, D., Perrier, H., Dorval, E. D., Martin, C., Bourgeois, H., Barthelemy, P. & Douillard, J. Y. (2001). Raltitrexed ("Tomudex") in the treatment of advanced pancreatic and biliary tract carcinomas: quality of life and efficacy results. *Proceedings of the American Society of Clinical Oncology* **20**, 147b (abstract 2339).

Fritz, P., Brambs, H. J., Schraube, P., Freund, U., Berns, C. & Wannenmacher, M. (1994). Combined external beam radiotherapy and intraluminal high dose rate brachytherapy on bile duct carcinomas. *International Journal of Radiation Oncology, Biology, Physics* **29**, 855–861.

Fulcher, A. S. & Turner, M. A. (2002). MR cholangiopancreatography. *Radiology Clinics of North America* **40**, 1363–1376.

Gallardo, J., Rubio, B., Fodor, M. & Ahumada, M. (2002). Gemcitabine in gallbladder cancer: clinical benefit assessment. *Proceedings of the American Society of Clinical Oncology* **21**, 123b (abstract 2305).

Gallardo, J. O., Rubio, B., Fodor, M., Orlandi, L., Yanez, M., Gamargo, C. & Ahumada, M. (2001). A phase II study of gemcitabine in gallbladder carcinoma. *Annals of Oncology* **12**, 1403–1406.

Gebbia, V., Giuliani, F., Maiello, E., Colucci, G., Verderame, F., Borsellino, N., Mauceri, G., Caruso, M., Tirrito, M. L. & Valdesi, M. (2001). Treatment of inoperable and/or metastatic biliary tree carcinomas with single-agent gemcitabine or in combination with levofolinic acid and infusional fluorouracil: results of a multicenter phase II study. *Journal of Clinical Oncology* **19**, 4089–4091.

Gebbia, V., Majello, E., Testa, A., Pezzella, G., Giuseppe, S., Giotta, F., Riccardi, F., Fortunato, S., Colucci, G. & Gebbia, N. (1996). Treatment of advanced adenocarcinomas of the exocrine pancreas and the gallbladder with 5-fluorouracil, high dose levofolinic acid and oral hydroxyurea on a weekly schedule. Results of a multicenter study of the Southern Italy Oncology Group (G.O.I.M.). *Cancer* **78**, 1300–1307.

Glimelius, B., Hoffman, K., Sjoden, P. O., Jacobsson, G., Sellstrom, H., Enander, L. K., Linne, T. & Svensson, C. (1996). Chemotherapy improves survival and quality of life in advanced pancreatic and biliary cancer. *Annals of Oncology* **7**, 593–600.

Gonzalez Gonzalez, D., Gouma, D. J., Rauws, E. A., van Gulik, T. M., Bosma, A. & Koedooder, C. (1999). Role of radiotherapy, in particular intraluminal brachytherapy, in the treatment of proximal bile duct carcinoma. *Annals of Oncology* **10**, 215–220.

Hann, L.E., Greatrex, K.V., Bach, A.M., Fong, Y. & Blumgart, L.H. (1997). Cholangiocarcinoma at the hepatic hilus: sonographic findings. *American Journal of Roentgenology* **168**, 985–989.

Harvey, J. H., Smith, F. P. & Schein, P. S. (1984). 5-Fluorouracil, mitomycin, and doxorubicin (FAM) in carcinoma of the biliary tract. *Journal of Clinical Oncology* **2**, 1245–1248.

Hsue, V., Wong, C. S., Moore, M., Erlichman, C., Cummings, B. J. & MacLeod, M. (1996). A phase I study of combined radiation therapy with 5-fluorouracil and low dose folinic acid in patients with locally advanced pancreatic or biliary carcinoma. *International Journal of Radiation Oncology, Biology, Physics* **34**, 445–450.

Hultcrantz, R., Olsson, R., Danielsson, A., Jarnerot, G., Loof, L., Ryden, B. O., Wahren, B. & Broome, U. (1999). A 3-year prospective study on serum tumor markers used for detecting cholangiocarcinoma in patients with primary sclerosing cholangitis. *Journal of Hepatology* **30**, 669–673.

Iwasaki, Y., Todoroki, T., Fukao, K., Ohara, K., Okamura, T. & Nishimura, A. (1988). The role of intraoperative radiation therapy in the treatment of bile duct cancer. *World Journal of Surgery* **12**, 91–98.

Jalanko, H., Kuusela, P., Roberts, P., Sipponen, P., Haglund, C. A. & Makela, O. (1984). Comparison of a new tumour marker, CA 19-9, with alpha-fetoprotein and carcinoembryonic antigen in patients with upper gastrointestinal diseases. *Journal of Clinical Pathology* **37**, 218–222.

Jani, C. R., Bhargava, P., Stuart, K. E., Rocha Lima, C. M. S., O'Donnell, J. L. & Savarese, D. M. F. (2002). Multicentre phase II trial of gemcitabine and irinotecan in patients with advanced or metastatic biliary cancer. *Proceedings of the American Society of Clinical Oncology* **21**, 125b (abstract 2313).

Johnson, D. W., Safai, C. & Goffinet, D. R. (1985). Malignant obstructive jaundice: treatment with external-beam and intracavitary radiotherapy. *International Journal of Radiation Oncology, Biology, Physics* **11**, 411–416.

Jones, D. V. Jr, Lozano, R., Hoque, A., Markowitz, A. & Patt, Y. Z. (1996). Phase II study of paclitaxel therapy for unresectable biliary tree carcinomas. *Journal of Clinical Oncology* **14**, 2306–2310.

Kajanti, M. & Pyrhonen, S. (1994). Epirubicin-sequential methotrexate-5-fluorouracil-leucovorin treatment in advanced cancer of the extrahepatic biliary system. A phase II study. *American Journal of Clinical Oncology* **17**, 223–226.

Karani, J., Fletcher, M., Brinkley, D., Dawson, J. L., Williams, R. & Nunnerley, H. (1985). Internal biliary drainage and local radiotherapy with iridium-192 wire in treatment of hilar cholangiocarcinoma. *Clinical Radiology* **36**, 603–606.

Kim, T. W., Ahn, J. H., Chang, H. M., Kim, J. H., Lee, J., Kim, M. W. & Kang, Y.-K. (2002). A phase II trial of capecitabine and cisplatin in previously untreated advanced biliary cancer. *Proceedings of the American Society of Clinical Oncology* **21**, 115b (abstr 2273).

Klatskin, G. (1965). Adenocarcinoma of the hepatic duct at its bifurcation within the porta hepatis: an unusual tumour with distinctive clinical and pathological features. *American Journal of Medicine* **38**, 241–256.

Klempnauer, J., Ridder, G. J., Werner, M., Weimann, A. & Pichlmayr, R. (1997). What constitutes long-term survival after surgery for hilar cholangiocarcinoma? *Cancer* **79**, 26–34.

Kopelson, G., Harisiadis, L., Tretter, P. & Chang, C. H. (1977). The role of radiation therapy in cancer of the extra-hepatic biliary system: an analysis of thirteen patients and a review of the literature of the effectiveness of surgery, chemotherapy and radiotherapy. *International Journal of Radiation Oncology, Biology, Physics* **2**, 883–894.

Koyama, K., Tanaka, J., Sato, Y., Seki, H., Kato, Y. & Umezawa, A. (1993). Experience in twenty patients with carcinoma of hilar bile duct treated by resection, targeting chemotherapy and intracavitary irradiation. *Surgical Gynecology and Obstetrics* **176**, 239–245.

Kubicka, S., Rudolph, K .L., Tietze, M. K., Lorenz, M. & Manns, M. (2001). Phase II study of systemic gemcitabine chemotherapy for advanced unresectable hepatobiliary carcinomas. *Hepatogastroenterology*, **48**, 783–789.

Kuhn, R., Ridwelski, K., Eichelmann, K., Fahlke, J., Hribaschek, A. & Lippert, H. (2001). Outpatient combination chemotherapy with gemcitabine and docetaxel in patients with cancer of the biliary system. *Proceedings of the American Society of Clinical Oncology* **20**, 130b (abstr 2272).

Kurathong, S., Lerdverasirikul, P., Wongpaitoon, V., Pramoolsinsap, C., Kanjanapitak, A., Varavithya, W., Phuapradit, P., Bunyaratvej, S., Upatham, E. S. & Brockelman, W. Y. (1985). Opisthorchis viverrini infection and cholangiocarcinoma. A prospective, case-controlled study. *Gastroenterology*, **89**, 151–156.

Lozano, R. D., Patt, Y. Z., Hassan, M. M., Frome, A., Vauthey, J. N., Ellis, L. M., Schnirer, I., Brown, T. D., Abbruzzese, J. L., Wolff, R. A. & Charnsangavej, C. (2000). Oral capecitabine (Xeloda) for the treatment of hepatobiliary cancers (hepatocellular carcinoma, cholangiocarcinoma, and gallbladder cancer). *Proceedings of the American Society of Clinical Oncology* **19**, 264a (abstract).

Lu, J. J., Bains, Y. S., Abdel-Wahab, M., Brandon, A. H., Wolfson, A. H., Raub, W. A., Wilkinson, C. M. & Markoe, A. M. (2002). High-dose-rate remote afterloading intracavitary brachytherapy for the treatment of extrahepatic biliary duct carcinoma. *Cancer Journal* **8**, 74–78.

Madariaga, J. R., Iwatsuki, S., Todo, S., Lee, R. G., Irish, W. & Starzl, T. E. (1998). Liver resection for hilar and peripheral cholangiocarcinomas: a study of 62 cases. *Annals of Surgery* **227**, 70–79.

Makela, J. T. & Kairaluoma, M. I. (1993). Superselective intra-arterial chemotherapy with mitomycin for gallbladder cancer. *British Journal of Surgery* **80**, 912–915.

Mani, S., Sciortino, D., Samuels, B., Arrietta, R., Schilsky, R.L., Vokes, E.E. & Benner, S. (1999). Phase II trial of uracil/tegafur (UFT) plus leucovorin in patients with advanced biliary carcinoma. *Investigational New Drugs* **17**, 97–101.

Mehta, V. K., Fisher, G. A., Ford, J. M., Poen, J. C., Vierra, M. A., Oberhelman, H. A. & Bastidas, A. J. (2001). Adjuvant chemoradiotherapy for "unfavourable" carcinoma of the ampulla of Vater: preliminary report. *Archives of Surgery* **136**, 65–69.

Meyers, W. C. & Jones, R. S. (1988). Internal radiation for bile duct cancer. *World Journal of Surgery* **12**, 99–104.

Mezawa, S., Homma, H., Sato, T., Doi, T., Miyanishi, K., Takada, K., Kukitsu, T., Murase, K., Yoshizaki, N., Takahashi, M., Sakamaki, S. & Niitsu, Y. (2000). A study of carboplatin-coated tube for the unresectable cholangiocarcinoma. *Hepatology* **32**, 916–923.

Mezger, J., Sauerbruch, T., Ko, Y., Wolter, H. & Funk, C. (1997). Phase II trial of gemcitabine (Gem) in biliary tract cancers (BTC). *Proceedings of the American Society of Clinical Oncology* **16**, 297a (abstract 1059).

Miller, R. L., Bowen, K. E. & Chun, H. G. (2002). A phase II study of liposomal doxorubicin (LD, Doxil) in patients with advanced hepatocellular carcinoma (HCC) or cholangiocarcinoma (CC). *Proceedings of the American Society of Clinical Oncology* **21**, 128b (abstract 2324).

Minsky, B. D., Kemeny, N., Armstrong, J. G., Reichman, B. & Botet, J. (1991). Extrahepatic biliary system cancer: an update of a combined modality approach. *American Journal of Clinical Oncology* **14**, 433–437.

Mitry, E., van Custem, E., Van Laethem, J., Gress, T., Jeziorski, K., Wagener, T., Reuse, S., Baron, B., Nordlinger, B. & Ducreux, M. (2002). A randomised phase II trial of weekly high-dose 5FU with and without folinic acid and cisplatin in patients with advanced biliary tract adenocarcinoma: the EORTC 40955 trial. *Proceedings of the American Society of Clinical Oncology* **21**, 175a (abstract 696).

Mittal, B., Deutsch, M. & Iwatsuki, S. (1985). Primary cancers of extrahepatic biliary passages. *International Journal of Radiation Oncology, Biology, Physics* **11**, 849–854.

Nakeeb, A., Pitt, H. A., Sohn, T. A., Coleman, J., Abrams, R. A., Piantadosi, S., Hruban, R. H., Lillemoe, K. D., Yeo, C. J. & Cameron, J. L. (1996). Cholangiocarcinoma. A spectrum of intrahepatic, perihilar, and distal tumors. *Annals of Surgery* **224**, 463–473; discussion 473–475.

Okada, S., Ishii, H., Nose, H., Yoshimori, M., Okusaka, T., Aoki, K., Iwasaki, M., Furuse, J. & Yoshino, M. (1994). A phase II study of cisplatin in patients with biliary tract carcinoma. *Oncology* **51**, 515–517.

Okada, S., Okusaka, T., Ishii, H., Ikeda, K., Nakasuka, H., Nakayama, F., Nagahama, H., Yoshimori, M., Iwasaki, M., Furuse, J., Yoshino, M., Miyaji, M. & Hoshino, M. (1997). Phase II trial of cisplatin, epirubicin and continuous infusion 5-fluorouracil (CEF therapy) for advanced gallbladder cancer (GBC). *Proceedings of the American Society of Clinical Oncology* **16**, 301a (abstract 1072).

Pahernik, S. A., Dellian, M., Berr, F., Tannapfel, A., Wittekind, C. & Goetz, A. E. (1998). Distribution and pharmacokinetics of Photofrin in human bile duct cancer. *Journal of Photochemistry and Photobiology B* **47**, 58–62.

Papakostas, P., Kouroussis, C., Androulakis, N., Samelis, G., Aravantinos, G., Kalbakis, K., Sarra, E., Souglakos, J., Kakolyris, S. & Georgoulias, V. (2001). First-line chemotherapy with docetaxel for unresectable or metastatic carcinoma of the biliary tract. A multicentre phase II study. *European Journal of Cancer* **37**, 1833–1838.

Patt, Y. Z., Hassan, M. M., Lozano, R. D., Waugh, K. A., Hoque, A. M., Frome, A. I., Lahoti, S., Ellis, L., Vauthey, J. N., Curley, S. A., Schnirer, I. I. & Raijman, I. (2001). Phase II trial of cisplatin, interferon alpha-2b, doxorubicin, and 5- fluorouracil for biliary tract cancer. *Clinical Cancer Research* **7**, 3375–3380.

Patt, Y. Z., Jones, D. V. Jr, Hoque, A., Lozano, R., Markowitz, A., Raijman, I., Lynch, P. & Charnsangavej, C. (1996). Phase II trial of intravenous flourouracil and subcutaneous interferon alfa-2b for biliary tract cancer. *Journal of Clinical Oncology* **14**, 2311–2315.

Pazdur, R., Royce, M. E., Rodriguez, G. I., Rinaldi, D. A., Patt, Y. Z., Hoff, P. M. & Burris, H. A. (1999). Phase II trial of docetaxel for cholangiocarcinoma. *American Journal of Clinical Oncology* **22**, 78–81.

Penz, M., Kornek, G. V., Raderer, M., Ulrich-Pur, H., Fiebiger, W., Lenauer, A., Depisch, D., Krauss, G., Schneeweiss, B. & Scheithauer, W. (2001). Phase II trial of two-weekly gemcitabine in patients with advanced biliary tract cancer. *Annals of Oncology* **12**, 183–186.

Pitt, H. A., Nakeeb, A., Abrams, R. A., Coleman, J., Piantadosi, S., Yeo, C. J., Lillemore, K. D. & Cameron, J. L. (1995). Perihilar cholangiocarcinoma. Postoperative radiotherapy does not improve survival. *Annals of Surgery* **221**, 788–797; discussion 797–798.

Quinn, M., Babb, P., Brock, A., Kirby, L. & Jones, J. (2001). Cancer Trends in England and Wales 1950–1999. London: The Stationery Office (Office for National Statistics).

Raderer, M., Hejna, M. H., Valencak, J. B., Kornek, G. V., Weinlander, G. S., Bareck, E., Lenauer, J., Brodowicz, T., Lang, F. & Scheithauer, W. (1999). Two consecutive phase II studies of 5-fluorouracil/leucovorin/mitomycin C and of gemcitabine in patients with advanced biliary cancer. *Oncology* **56**, 177–180.

Ravry, M. J., Omura, G. A., Bartolucci, A. A., Einhorn, L., Kramer, B. & Davila, E. (1986). Phase II evaluation of cisplatin in advanced hepatocellular carcinoma and cholangiocarcinoma: a Southeastern Cancer Study Group Trial. *Cancer Treatment Reports* **70**, 311–312.

Reding, R., Buard, J. L., Lebeau, G. & Launois, B. (1991). Surgical management of 552 carcinomas of the extrahepatic bile ducts (gallbladder and periampullary tumors excluded). Results of the French Surgical Association Survey. *Annals of Surgery* **213**, 236–241.

Robertson, J. M., McGinn, C. J., Walker, S., Marx, M. V., Kessler, M. L., Ensminger, W. D. & Lawrence, T. S. (1997). A phase I trial of hepatic arterial bromodeoxyuridine and conformal radiation therapy for patients with primary hepatobiliary cancers or colorectal liver metastases. *International Journal of Radiation Oncology, Biology, Physics* **39**, 1087–1092.

Rosen, C. B., Nagorney, D. M., Wiesner, R. H., Coffey, R. J. Jr & LaRusso, N. F. (1991). Cholangiocarcinoma complicating primary sclerosing cholangitis. *Annals of Surgery* **213**, 21–25.

Rumalla, A., Baron, T. H., Wang, K. K., Gores, G. J., Stadheim, L. M. & de Groen, P. C. (2001). Endoscopic application of photodynamic therapy for cholangiocarcinoma. *Gastrointestinal Endoscopy* **53**, 500–504.

Sanz-Altamira, P. M., Ferrante, K., Jenkins, R. L., Lewis, W. D., Huberman, M. S. & Stuart, K. E. (1998). A phase II trial of 5-fluorouracil, leucovorin, and carboplatin in patients with unresectable biliary tree carcinoma. *Cancer* **82**, 2321–2325.

Schima, W., Prokesch, R., Osterreicher, C., Thurnher, S., Fugger, R., Schofl, R., Havelec, L. & Lammer, J. (1997). Biliary Wallstent endoprosthesis in malignant hilar obstruction: long-term results with regard to the type of obstruction. *Clinical Radiology* **52**, 213–219.

Schwartz, D. A. (1986). Cholangiocarcinoma associated with liver fluke infection: a preventable source of morbidity in Asian immigrants. *American Journal of Gastroenterology* **81**, 76–79.

Shiina, T., Mikuriya, S., Uno, T., Toita, T., Serizawa, S., Itami, J., Kawai, S. & Tani, M. (1992). Radiotherapy of cholangiocarcinoma: the roles for primary and adjuvant therapies. *Cancer Chemotherapy and Pharmacology* **31**, S115–S118.

Smith, G. W., Bukowski, R. M., Hewlett, J. S. & Groppe, C. W. (1984). Hepatic artery infusion of 5-fluorouracil and mitomycin C in cholangiocarcinoma and gallbladder carcinoma. *Cancer*, **54**, 1513–1516.

Smoron, G. L. (1977). Radiation therapy of carcinoma of gallbladder and biliary tract. *Cancer* **40**, 1422–1424.

Sumiyoshi, K., Nagai, E., Chijiiwa, K. & Nakayama, F. (1991). Pathology of carcinoma of the gallbladder. *World Journal of Surgery* **15**, 315–321.

Taal, B. G., Audisio, R. A., Bleiberg, H., Blijham, G. H., Neijt, J. P., Veenhof, C. H., Duez, N. & Sahmoud, T. (1993). Phase II trial of mitomycin C (MMC) in advanced gallbladder and biliary tree carcinoma. An EORTC Gastrointestinal Tract Cancer Cooperative Group Study. *Annals of Oncology* **4**, 607–609.

Taieb, J., Mitry, E., Boige, V., Artru, P., Ezenfis, J., Lecomte, T., Clavero-Fabri, M. C., Vaillant, J. N., Rougier, P. & Ducreux, M. (2002). Optimization of 5-fluorouracil (5-FU)/cisplatin combination chemotherapy with a new schedule of leucovorin, 5-FU and cisplatin (LV5FU2-P regimen) in patients with biliary tract carcinoma. *Annals of Oncology* **13**, 1192–1196.

Takada, T., Nimura, Y., Katoh, H., Nagakawa, T., Nakayama, T., Matsushiro, T., Amano, H. & Wada, K. (1998). Prospective randomized trial of 5-fluorouracil, doxorubicin, and mitomycin C for non-resectable pancreatic and biliary carcinoma: multicenter randomized trial. *Hepatogastroenterology* **45**, 2020–2026.

Tillich, M., Mischinger, H. J., Preisegger, K. H., Rabl, H. & Szolar, D. H. (1998). Multiphasic helical CT in diagnosis and staging of hilar cholangiocarcinoma. *American Journal of Roentgenology* **171**, 651–658.

Todoroki, T., Iwasaki, Y., Orii, K., Otsuka, M., Ohara, K., Kawamoto, T. & Nakamura, K. (1991). Resection combined with intraoperative radiation therapy (IORT) for stage IV (TNM) gallbladder carcinoma. *World Journal of Surgery* **15**, 357–366.

Treadwell, T. A. & Hardin, W. J. (1976). Primary carcinoma of the gallbladder. The role of adjunctive therapy in its treatment. *American Journal of Surgery* **132**, 703–706.

Urego, M., Flickinger, J. C. & Carr, B. I. (1999). Radiotherapy and multimodality management of cholangiocarcinoma. *International Journal of Radiation Oncology, Biology, Physics* **44**, 121–126.

Vaittinen, E. (1970). Carcinoma of the gall-bladder. A study of 390 cases diagnosed in Finland 1953–1967. *Annales Chirurgiae et Gynaecologiae Fennica Supplementum* **168**, 1–81.

Van Laethem, J. L., Deviere, J., Bourgeois, N., Love, J., Gelin, M., Cremer, M. & Adler, M. (1995). Cholangiographic findings in deteriorating primary sclerosing cholangitis. *Endoscopy* **27**, 223–228.

Verderame, F., Mandina, P., Abruzzo, F., Scarpulla, M. & Di Leo, R. (2000). Biliary tract cancer: our experience with gemcitabine treatment. *Anticancer Drugs* **11**, 707–708.

Weinbren, K. & Mutum, S. S. (1983). Pathological aspects of cholangiocarcinoma. *Journal of Pathology* **139**, 217–238.

Weissmann, A. & Ludwig, H. (1999). Intraarterial gemcitabine for treatment of inoperable pancreatic and cholangiocarcinoma. *Proceedings of the American Society of Clinical Oncology* **18**, 305a (abstract).

Whittington, R., Neuberg, D., Tester, W. J., Benson, A. B. III & Haller, D. G. (1995). Protracted intravenous fluorouracil infusion with radiation therapy in the management of localized pancreaticobiliary carcinoma: a phase I Eastern Cooperative Oncology Group Trial. *Journal of Clinical Oncology* **13**, 227–232.

Wolkov, H. B., Graves, G. M., Won, M., Sause, W. T., Byhardt, R. W. & Hanks, G. E. (1992). Intraoperative radiation therapy of extrahepatic biliary carcinoma: a report of RTOG-8506. *American Journal of Clinical Oncology* **15**, 323–327.

Yamamoto, M., Takasaki, K., Yoshikawa, T., Ueno, K. & Nakano, M. (1998). Does gross appearance indicate prognosis in intrahepatic cholangiocarcinoma? *Journal of Surgical Oncology* **69**, 162–167.

Zatonski, W. A., Lowenfels, A. B., Boyle, P., Maisonneuve, P., Bueno de Mesquita, H. B., Ghadirian, P., Jain, M., Przewozniak, K., Baghurst, P., Moerman, C. J., Simard, A., Howe, G. R., McMichael, A. J., Hsieh, C. C. & Walker, A. M. (1997). Epidemiologic aspects of gallbladder cancer: a case–control study of the SEARCH Program of the International Agency for Research on Cancer. *Journal of the National Cancer Institute* **89**, 1132–1138.

Zoepf, T., Jakobs, R., Arnold, J. C., Apel, D., Rosenbaum, A. & Riemann, J. F. (2001a). Photodynamic therapy for palliation of non-resectable bile duct cancer – preliminary results with a new diode laser system. *American Journal of Gastroenterology* **96**, 2093–2097.

Zoepf, T., Jakobs, R., Rosenbaum, A., Apel, D., Arnold, J. C. & Riemann, J. F. (2001b). Photodynamic therapy with 5-aminolevulinic acid is not effective in bile duct cancer. *Gastrointestinal Endoscopy* **54**, 763–766.

PART 4

Clinical governance of upper gastrointestinal cancer services

Generating scientific evidence for the management of upper gastrointestinal malignancy: the role of the Cochrane Collaboration

Chris Williams

Introduction

The use of explicit, systematic methods in reviews limits bias (systematic errors) and reduces chance effects by increasing the number of participants, thus providing more reliable results upon which to draw conclusions and make decisions (Antman 1992). Systematic reviews can establish where effects of healthcare are consistent, can be applied across populations and in different settings. They can also show where effects may vary significantly.

Meta-analysis, the use of statistical methods to summarise the results of independent studies, can provide more precise estimates of the effects of healthcare than those derived from the individual studies included in a systematic review (L'Abbe 1987; Sacks 1987; Thacker 1988). Systematic reviews ideally include meta-analysis, but often this is not possible because the questions, trial populations and method of delivering therapy were too variable to allow meaningful pooling of results in a meta-analysis.

Recognition of the key role of reviews in synthesising and disseminating the results of research has prompted people to consider the validity of narrative reviews. Social science and psychology led this field and it was not until the late 1980s that people drew attention to the poor scientific quality of healthcare review articles (Mulrow 1987; Yusuf 1987; Oxman 1988). The first survey of the quality of narrative reviews in cancer was not published until 1997.

Why do we need reviews?

Apart from the need to find time-efficient means of using the literature to help make decisions, there is good evidence that a systematic approach can produce results that change practice. Systematic reviews of therapy for acute myocardial infarction (Antman 1992) show how careful review of all of the evidence can change thinking. Early experience with thrombolytic therapy was largely ignored and narrative reviews and textbooks failed to routinely recommend such treatment for 10–15 years after meta-analysis would have shown these treatments to be effective. Conversely, lignocaine (lidocaine) has been consistently recommended for use in myocardial infarction (MI) by narrative reviews and textbooks, when there was no evidence of benefit. Thus, systematic reviews could, in this situation, change practice and help researchers to develop new trials.

Reviews are useful because they:
1 are an efficient use of time;
2 can help support individual patient decisions;
3 can help in preparing guidelines and treatment protocols;
4 can help in developing and planning new clinical research.

What is wrong with narrative reviews?

Reviews are not new, so what is wrong with the classical or narrative review that has been used for many generations? Mulrow (1987) was the first to examine the methodological quality of narrative reviews in general medicine. Since then, several similar studies have examined the methods used in different branches of medicine, including cancer. The findings have been uniformly similar. Bramwell & Williams (1997) reported on the methodological quality of reviews published in the *Journal of Clinical Oncology* from its inception in 1983 through to 1995. In the areas that are regarded as key to reducing the risk of bias (data identification, selection of data to be included, assessment of the validity of that data, quantitative synthesis of the data), fewer than 10% of the reviews used methods designed to reduce bias.

What are the main elements of a systematic review?

Systematic reviews aim to address the weaknesses identified in narrative reviews by paying careful attention to those areas where bias may be evident in the process of finding, selecting, extracting data from and synthesising the results of trials asking similar questions. This essentially means writing a protocol setting out how the review is to be performed to minimise bias. The key steps in preparing a systematic review are briefly discussed in the following sections. Users of systematic reviews should be looking to see if the reviewers have done a thorough job in each of these areas.

1. Locating and selecting studies

A comprehensive, unbiased search of the literature is one of the key differences between a systematic review and a narrative review. To reduce the risk of bias it is important to use a variety of sources to identify studies and to have a systematic approach to selecting studies for inclusion in a review. The potential for reference bias (a tendency to preferentially cite studies supporting one's own views) is reduced by using multiple search strategies.(Gotzsche 1987; Ravnskov 1992). It should also be remembered that strongly 'positive' trials are more likely to be published on multiple occasions, sometimes with different authors and different results (Tramer 1997).

2. Quality assessment of studies

Quality assessment of individual studies summarised in a systematic review is required to:

1 limit bias in conducting the systematic review;
2 gain insight into potential comparisons;
3 guide interpretation of findings.

This quality assessment should look at those factors related to:

1 applicability of the findings: also called external validity or generalisability. This is related to the definition of the key components of the question being addressed. Specifically, whether the findings of the trial are applicable to a particular population, intervention strategy and how the people, interventions and outcomes of interest were defined by these studies and the reviewers.
2 validity of individual studies: interpretation of results is dependent upon the validity of the included studies which is addressed in more detail in the next sections.

3. Validity

When preparing or reading a systematic review (or trial report), the validity of an individual study is the extent to which its design and conduct are likely to prevent systematic errors, or bias (Moher 1995). An issue that should not be confused with validity is precision. Precision is a measure of the likelihood of chance effects leading to random errors. It is reflected in the confidence interval around the estimate of effect from each study and the weight given to the results of each study when an overall estimate of effect or weighted average is derived. Thus more precise results are given more weight.

Variation in validity can explain variation in the results of the studies included in a systematic review. More rigorous studies designed to avoid bias should be more likely to yield results that are closer to the 'truth'. Quantitative analysis of results from studies with varying degrees of validity can result in 'false positive' conclusions if the less rigorous studies are biased toward overestimating treatment effectiveness. They can also come to 'false negative' conclusions if less rigorous studies are biased towards underestimating an intervention's effect (Detsky 1992).

4. Sources of bias in trials of healthcare interventions

There are four sources of systematic bias (see figure below) in trials of healthcare:

1 selection bias;
2 performance bias;
3 attrition bias;
4 detection bias.

Unfortunately, we do not have strong empirical evidence of a relationship between trial outcomes and the risk of these biases (Moher 1995, 1996b), but there is a logical basis for suspecting such relationships and good reason to consider these potential biases when assessing studies for a review (Feinstein 1985).

Role of the Cochrane Collaboration

The Cochrane Collaboration is an international body that prepares and maintains systematic reviews of interventions in all areas of healthcare. It has about 8,000 contributors, most of whom are volunteers. The key groups in Cochrane are the Collaborative Review Groups, who support the reviewers in their work in preparing and maintaining reviews. The Cochrane Upper Gastro-intestinal and Pancreatic Diseases review group is based in Leeds, UK. The Co-ordinating editor is Professor David Forman and the Review Group Co-ordinator is Janet Lilleyman. The review group's e-mail address and web-site addresses are cochrane@leeds.ac.uk and http://cochrane.leeds.ac.uk, respectively.

Currently (July 2004) the output of the review group was:
- 16 published reviews (5 cancer);
- 30 published protocols (11 cancer), with review in preparation;
- 17 registered titles (4 cancer), with protocol in preparation.

There is a clear need to increase the number of reviews to ensure that they cover the main questions in this area of medicine.

Cochrane has a clear and detailed methodology for preparing reviews that is designed to ensure that the quality is as high as possible. There is editorial input in the design of the question, preparation of the protocol (the background and methods section of the eventual review) as well as at completion of the review. There is also external peer review of the protocol and final review.

Using these processes the Upper Gastro-intestinal and Pancreatic Diseases review group have produced the following cancer reviews:
1 Post-operative radiotherapy for oesophageal cancer.
2 Pre-operative chemotherapy for resectable oesophageal cancer.
3 Chemotherapy and radiotherapy without surgery versus radiotherapy alone for localised oesophageal cancer.
4 Extended versus limited surgery for gastric cancer.

Protocols of cancer reviews in preparation include:
1 Chemotherapy and radiotherapy for pancreatic cancer.
2 Post-operative radiotherapy for oesophageal cancer.
3 Enteral versus parenteral nutrition for upper GI cancer.
4 Chemotherapy for advanced gastric cancer.
5 Pharmacological and endoscopic therapies for Barrett's oesophagus.

6   Transthoracic resection for oesophageal cancer.
7   Chemotherapy for metastatic carcinoma of the oesophagus and gastric cardia.
8   Stent versus surgery for palliation of pancreatic cancer.
9   Endoscopic mucosal resection for early gastric cancer.

Among the many potential reviews in this area, the review group have given high priority to finding reviewers interested in preparing the following reviews:
1   surgery for pancreatic cancer;
2   intra-peritoneal chemotherapy for gastric cancer;
3   stent of photodynamic therapy for oesophageal cancer;
4   infection management during chemotherapy.

Potential reviewers may review any of the topics within the scope of the review group. This includes prevention, screening, primary therapy, palliative therapy, issues of quality of life/symptom control, psycho-social issues, delivery of care and many other topics. The only area that is clearly 'off limits' is that of diagnosis. At present, the quality of primary diagnostic research is very variable and there is no reliable methodology for pooling data from the traditional types of diagnostic study. The Cochrane Collaboration is, however, working to overcome these problems and is likely to include diagnostic tests in its future review topics.

Conclusion

The Cochrane Upper Gastro-intestinal and Pancreatic Diseases review group is looking for reviewers, peer referees, and journal hand-searchers. The group will give support in training, software, literature searching, trial identification and statistics. Any reader interested in working with the group should contact them at cochrane@leeds.ac.uk.

Systematic reviews can sometimes be helpful in deciding on the treatment of individual patients, but their role at the moment is probably more to help guideline producers and researchers designing new trials. Most reviews in cancer do not give a clear unequivocal answer that can be used to guide therapeutic decisions, and there are currently many gaps where there are no systematic reviews. However, the degree of uncertainty around a specific question where there is a systematic review may be helpful when formulating guidelines and is invaluable in summarising the literature and planning the next research steps.

Researchers should bear in mind that there are multiple points in clinical practice where decisions are made. Many of these are not the major treatment decisions (adjuvant chemotherapy after surgery, for instance), but are still important and have a major effect on the patient and their family as well as on the practice of medicine. Issues such as follow up (Jeffery 2003), how best to deliver care (Lewin 2003; Thompson 2003), how to communicate better (Scott 2003; Edwards 2003), etc., are often forgotten while we wrestle over issues important to clinicians. Despite a lack of evidence on some of these forgotten areas, clinicians and others routinely make decisions that have a major impact on the patient and hospital system.

References

Antman, E.M., Lau, J., Kupelnick, B., Mosteller, F. & Chalmers, T. C. (1992). A comparison of results of meta-analyses of randomized control trials and recommendations of clinical experts. Treatments for myocardial infarction. *Journal of the American Medical Association* **268**, 240–248.

Bramwell, V. H. C. & Williams C. J. (1997). Do authors of review articles use systematic methods to identify, assess and synthesize information? *Annals of Oncology* **8**, 1185–1196.

Detsky, A. S., Naylor, C. D., O'Rourke, K., McGreer, A. J. & L'Abbe, K. A. (1992). Incorporating variations in the quality of individual randomized trials into meta-analysis. *Journal of Clinical Epidemiology* **45**, 255–265.

Edwards, A., Unigwe, S., Elwyn, G. & Hood, K. (2003). Personalised risk communication for informed decision making about entering screening programs (Cochrane Review). In: *The Cochrane Library*, issue 1. Oxford: Update Software.

Feinstein, A. R. (1985). *Clinical Epidemiology: The Architecture of Clinical Research*, pp. 39–52. Philadelphia: Saunders.

Gotzsche, P. C. (1987). Reference bias in reports of drug trials. *British Medical Journal* **295**, 654–656.

Jeffery, G. M., Hickey, B. E. & Hider, P. (2003). Follow-up strategies for patients treated for non-metastatic colorectal cancer (Cochrane Review). In: *The Cochrane Library*, issue 1. Oxford: Update Software.

L'Abbe, K. A., Detsky, A. S. & O'Rourke, K. (1987). Meta-analysis in clinical research. *Annals of Internal Medicine* **107**, 224–233.

Lewin, S. A., Skea, Z. C., Entwistle, V., Zwarenstein, M. & Dick, J. (2003). Interventions for providers to promote a patient-centred approach in clinical consultations (Cochrane Review). In: *The Cochrane Library*, issue 1. Oxford: Update Software.

Moher, D., Jadad, A., Nichol, G., Penman, M., Tugwell, T. & Walsh, S. (1995). Assessing the quality of randomized controlled trials: an annotated bibliography of scales and checklists. *Controlled Clinical Trials* **16**, 62–73.

Moher, D., Jadad, A. R. & Tugwell, P. (1996). Assessing the quality of randomized controlled trials: current issues and future directions. *International Journal of Technology Assessment in Health Care* **12**, 195–208.

Mulrow, C. D. (1987). The medical review article: state of the science. *Annals of Internal Medicine* **106**, 485–488.

Oxman, A. D. & Guyatt, G. H. (1988). Guidelines for reading literature reviews. *Canadian Medical Association Journal* **138**, 697–703.

Ravnskov, U. (1992). Cholesterol lowering trials in coronary heart disease: frequency of citation and outcome. *British Medical Journal* **305**, 15–19.

Sacks, H. S., Berrier, J., Reitman, D., Ancona-Berk, V. A. & Chalmers, T. C. (1987). Meta-analyses of randomized controlled trials. *New England Journal of Medicine* **316**, 450–455.

Scott, J. T., Entwistle, V. A., Sowden, A. J. & Watt. I. (2003). Recordings or summaries of consultations for people with cancer (Cochrane Review). In: *The Cochrane Library*, issue 1. Oxford: Update Software.

Thacker, S. B. (1988). Meta-analysis: a quantitative approach to research integration. *Journal of the American Medical Association* **259**, 1685–1689.

Thomson O'Brien, M. A., Oxman, A. D., Davis, D. A., Haynes, R. B., Freemantle, N. & Harvey, E. L. (2003). Audit and feedback versus alternative strategies: effects on professional practice and health care outcomes (Cochrane Review). In: *The Cochrane Library*, issue 1. Oxford: Update Software.

Tramer, M. R., Reynolds, D. J., Moore, R. A. & McQuay, H. J. (1997). Impact of covert duplicate publication on meta-analysis: a case study. *British Medical Journal* **315**, 635–640.

Yusuf, S., Simon, R. & Ellenberg, S. (eds) (1987). Proceedings of "Methodologic issues in overviews of randomized clinical trials". *Statistics in Medicine* **6**, 217–409.

Chapter 13

Reorganisation and re-provision of clinical services for upper gastrointestinal cancer

William Allum

Introduction

The outcome for patients with upper gastrointestinal cancer has traditionally been poor. Symptomatic presentation has frequently been associated with advanced disease, limiting the treatment options to palliative interventions for the majority. Improvements in outcome, however, have been slowly but steadily evolving over the past 20 years as understanding of presentation, diagnostic techniques and treatment modalities has developed. To ensure all patients receive the appropriate management, reorganisation of services has occurred in some parts of the UK but unfortunately this has not been uniform, for a variety of reasons. Recent professionally developed and Government-supported initiatives are attempting to redress the balance to ensure equity of service delivery for all patients. These initiatives require significant resource, which is often considered a limiting factor. However, new methodologies to determine where service redesign can be implemented are beginning to make significant progress in overcoming particular bottlenecks in service provision. As a result, qualitative improvements in the way in which patients are managed are occurring.

Background

Cancers of the upper gastrointestinal tract accounted for 18,250 deaths in the UK in 1997 (Office for National Statistics 1999). Epidemiologically, there have been significant changes in the disease incidence. Gastric cancer was the commonest malignancy worldwide at the turn of the 20th century. However, changes in diet principally have resulted in a marked decrease in incidence over the past 40 years. In 1994, there were 9,780 new cases in the UK compared with 14,850 in 1962. This reduction in incidence has occurred during a period of migration of the site of disease towards the oesophago-gastric junction. As a result, cancers of the lower third of the oesophagus and oesophago-gastric junction are showing the most rapid rise in incidence of the common solid cancers. Incidence of carcinoma of the pancreas has begun to plateau after showing a steady rise after the mid-twentieth century.

Regional Cancer Registry data have been the principal source of outcome data in the past 50 years. A series of reviews undertaken at the West Midlands Cancer Registry for the period 1957–81 has provided a baseline against which current treatment outcomes can be compared (Matthews *et al.* 1987; Fielding *et al.* 1989; Bramhall *et al.* 1995). The overall 5-year survival and the 5-year survival after curative resection are shown in Table 13.1. The overall 5-year survival rates are extremely low, largely reflecting the late stage of disease at presentation. The few cases being eligible for curative resection confirms this: oesophagus 27%; stomach 20.8%; pancreas 2.6%. Indeed, despite curative resection, post-treatment survival is low.

Table 13.1 Upper gastrointestinal cancer 5-year survival 1957–81

	Overall (%)	Curative resection (%)
Oesophagus	3.8	15.7
Stomach	4.6	25.8
Pancreas	0.0	9.7

These results reflect the time when surgery was the only option for treatment. Non-surgical treatments of chemotherapy and radiotherapy, particularly in the adjuvant setting, were not established. Non-specialists undertook operations. Patients came through the system at varying rates and the need to combine treatments and investigative modalities was not fully appreciated.

Improvements in patient management

These limited results have naturally been a significant driver to develop methods of improving the results of treatment (Allum *et al.* 2002). Experience from Japan, where gastric cancer was a major public health problem in the 1960s, has provided a model for the West to follow. Screening programmes, standardisation of investigation, consistency of surgical technique and interdisciplinary team working have proved fundamental to the Japanese approach.

In the UK, the incidence of gastric cancer precludes screening programmes. However, several studies have reported success with early diagnostic interventions. For example, in Birmingham a study evaluated early endoscopy for those patients presenting to their general practitioner with dyspepsia. Over a 4-year period, 2,600 patients from a population of 100,000 were examined. Gastro-oesophageal cancer was diagnosed in 57 (2%) patients, with 12 (22%) having cancers limited to the mucosa and submucosa, early gastric cancer (Hallissey *et al.* 1990). This clearly demonstrated that improving access to diagnostic services resulted in diagnosis at an earlier stage.

Technological advances have had a significant effect on the assessment of disease at diagnosis, thus ensuring the most appropriate stage-related treatment. Spiral CT scanning has a reported accuracy for assessing the extent of a primary gastric cancer of 68–86%. The addition of laparoscopy has improved the diagnosis of small volume intra-abdominal disease, which is not apparent on cross-sectional imaging. More recently, endoscopic ultrasound has had a major effect on the assessment of the operability of oesophageal cancer, where again there are limitations for external scanning in the assessment of the thoracic oesophagus.

Approaches to treatment have changed with greater specialisation. The Leeds group have reported survival figures equivalent to the Japanese after electing to perform routinely an extended lymph-node dissection in gastric cancer surgery (Table 13. 2) (Sue-Ling *et al.*1993). Furthermore, a review of the UK pancreatic centres has shown how surgical outcome benefits from the concentration of pancreatic cancer surgery in those units seeing the largest volume of patients (Neoptolemos *et al*, 1997). Bachmann *et al.* (2002) have also demonstrated how outcome in gastro-oesophageal cancer improves with increased volume of activity not only for specialists but also for the hospitals in which they work.

Table 13.2 Five-year survival after D2 resection for gastric cancer (including operative mortality) (Sue-Ling *et al.* 1993)

Overall: 54%
Stage I: 87%
Stage II: 65%
Stage III: 24%

These representative examples are part of the evidence that has accumulated to demonstrate that it is possible to improve the outcome for patients with upper gastrointestinal cancers. Compilation of the evidence is time consuming and although enthusiasts have been demonstrating what can be achieved, such approaches have not been uniformly available. As a result, there have been a series of initiatives to attempt to spread these approaches throughout the NHS.

Calman–Hine recommendations

In 1995 the UK Chief Medical Officers (Department of Health and the Welsh Office 1995) published a policy document with a series of recommendations attempting to begin the process of improving cancer services nationally and ensuring equity of availability of high-quality care. The principal recommendations related to the organisation of services. It was proposed that cancers should be treated in designated cancer units, which were closely related to designated cancer centres. The key concept of these proposals was that of critical mass. A unit would be appropriately designated if it managed the number of patients considered to represent a critical mass. Where the numbers of a particular cancer were small, several units would refer such cases to the centre. In high-volume and very low-volume cancers, application of this concept is straightforward. However, in less common cancers such as upper gastrointestinal disease, this approach initially proved more difficult to implement. This is partly explained by the symptoms of upper gastrointestinal cancers significantly overlapping with those of benign disease and partly by patients presenting to the general gastroenterology service in such numbers that are considered not to warrant specialist referral.

The other principal but related recommendation was that multidisciplinary teams should manage cancers. This promoted the relationship between cancer centres and cancer units and has ensured that patients are managed by the appropriate disciplines. This initially also produced difficulties as there were limited numbers of oncologists to provide the necessary support for all cancers. In many places an oncologist from a centre would visit a unit, be responsible for a variety of cancers, yet would not necessarily be able to fully support the unit tumour site-specific teams.

National Cancer Plan (2000)

Although local commissioners of healthcare have used the Calman–Hine recommendations to change the delivery of cancer service, the relative lack of resource has made the process slow. In 2000 the National Cancer Plan was published (Department of Health 2000). This is a 10-year plan designed to radically change the way in which cancer care is provided (Table 13.3). Again, there are changes in the organisation of services, building on the Calman–Hine recommendations. An infrastructure of 34 cancer networks has been put in place throughout the country, and within each network there is a mechanism for all involved in the treatment of a specific cancer to contribute to developing the local service and be involved in setting the agenda for improvement. The plan was announced with an initial 3-year funding programme of £570 million, which was intended to resource the developments.

Table 13.3 Key issues of the National Cancer Plan 2000

Prevention
Screening
Community services
Waiting times for diagnosis and treatment
Improving outcomes of treatment
Improving quality of care
Manpower
Facilities
Research and development
Implementation

A series of targets have been set to ensure that patients have early access to diagnostic services, specialist opinion, investigation and specialist treatment (Table 13.4). Already, the two-week rule has enabled 98% of those whom the general practitioner believes may have cancer to be seen by a specialist within two weeks of referral.

Table 13.4 National Cancer Plan targets

Maximum two week wait from referral by general practitoner to specialist clinic.
Maximum one month wait from diagnosis to treatment for:

   breast cancer by 2001;

   all cancers by 2005.

Maximum two month wait from urgent GP referral to treatment for:

Breast cancer by 2002.

All cancers by 2005.

One month wait from urgent referral to treatment for all cancers by 2008.

In upper gastrointestinal cancer, the two-week rule initiative (Table 13.5) has caused some concern because of the lack of specificity of symptoms. In some centres the number of cancers diagnosed by the two-week rule has proven to be a small proportion of the total number of cancers seen. Most seem to present through a variety of other sources. Thus, although many patients with suspicious symptoms are being seen and diagnosed quickly, not many are found to have cancer. Furthermore, there is concern that those who have cancer but with less significant symptoms are being seen with a lesser priority.

Table 13.5 Referral guidelines for upper gastrointestinal symptoms under the two-week rule

Dysphagia

Dyspepsia with weight loss / anaemia / anorexia

Dyspepsia >55 years with high-risk features

Dyspepsia with family history / Barrett's / pernicious anaemia / previous peptic ulcer / known dysplasia, atrophic gastritis, intestinal metaplasia

Jaundice

Upper abdominal mass

Another key part of the National Cancer Plan is the development of Improving Outcomes Guidance for those commissioning cancer services. Appropriate clinical and non-clinical specialists have produced these guidance documents after careful evaluation of all the available evidence. This has enabled the production of a set of standards to which units and centres need to adhere so that the approach to a particular cancer can be constant throughout the country.

Improving Outcomes Guidance

The Improving Outcomes Guidance for upper gastrointestinal cancer was published in 2001 (Department of Health 2001). All aspects of oesophageal, gastric and pancreatic cancer including epidemiology, diagnosis, staging, treatment and organisation of service delivery have been assessed, and evidence-based recommendations have been produced. The key recommendations were that hospitals, which provide services for upper gastrointestinal cancer, should work together in an integrated cancer network. There should be documented local referral policies for diagnosis of upper gastrointestinal cancer, jointly agreed by all levels of service including primary care. Specialist oesophago-gastric cancer teams and pancreatic cancer teams, serving populations of over one million and two to four million, respectively, should be established at appropriate cancer centres and units. There should be clear documented policies agreed for patient referral between hospitals. Co-ordinated palliative support and specialist care should be available to all who need it. Finally, systems should be established to audit key processes and outcomes of treatment.

A core component is that specialist treatment is on a population basis. Thus existing cancer units that, for example, cover a population of 350,000, would be designated as local diagnostic units. Those patients diagnosed with cancer in such units would need to be transferred to their network centre for specialist treatment. This requires the development of a local team, which works closely within agreed protocol with the cancer centre specialist team.

A significant implication of this approach is the effect on upper gastrointestinal surgery. The effective centralisation of surgery raised considerable concerns among upper gastrointestinal surgeons over the delivery of upper gastrointestinal surgical services at the cancer units. The Association of Upper Gastrointestinal Surgeons of Great Britain and Ireland undertook a survey of their membership to evaluate these concerns. The main areas of contention were the provision of services according to the populations cited in the guidance and the concept that the related increased volume of activity would translate into improved outcome. It was felt that a population of 500,000 for oeosphago-gastric cancer would be more pragmatic, not only to deliver specialist surgery but also to ensure appropriate upper gastrointestinal expertise for benign work. It was also argued that the minimum number of resections per surgeon per year should be 6–10, which would be achievable within units serving this population. For pancreatic cancer it was recognised that there would need to be centralisation. However, again a smaller population base of 1.5 million would provide sufficient surgical activity for a two-surgeon unit. The lack of information technology support within most units was an additional area of concern particularly because of the negative effect on data recording and evidence of outcome.

Appropriate representations have been made about these concerns. The process of implementation of the guidance, however, is planned to continue. Individual units and centres are undergoing peer review against the set of standards derived from the guidance. Action plans from individual networks are under development so that implementation can occur. Although these plans can have interim arrangements, it is anticipated that centralisation of the surgical procedures will be in place according to the guidance populations by the end of 2005. An issue of concern relates to the provision of resources for the associated changes. Commissioners of healthcare have a limited resource and by necessity undertake priority setting to meet a spectrum of targets, not all related to cancer. The rates of progress towards the 2005 target are likely to be variable across the country, even though the aim is to reach a standard of approach irrespective of where in the UK a patient presents.

Although most of the controversy over the guidance has concentrated on the surgical aspects, there are many other parts of the total patient journey, which need careful consideration. Attention to these issues has resulted in a thorough reconsideration of how the service is delivered. To facilitate service reorganisation and to address some of the concerns related to commissioning, there has been considerable interest in the redesign methodologies of the Cancer Services Collaborative.

Cancer Services Collaborative

The Cancer Services Collaborative (CSC), launched in 1999, has become a major component of the NHS Modernisation Agency. It has developed from a series of projects looking at ways of improving the experience of patients with cancer from a variety of perspectives. The aims of the CSC are to provide certainty and choice for patients, to pre-plan and pre-schedule care at timings to suit patients and to reduce unnecessary delays and restrictions on access. In addition, patient and carer satisfaction is an important goal achieved by providing a personalised consistent service. Finally, it is intended that the patient should receive the best care in the best place by the best person/team. The initiatives of redesigning service provision are now well established and are now a key component of service improvement.

There are two principal approaches which are fundamental to CSC redesign. Firstly, there is the assessment of the demand for a service and definition of the capacity of the unit to deliver the service. Secondly, there is the process of mapping where details of the patient journey are evaluated by all involved to allow identification of 'bottlenecks' and to determine whether additional resource or change in working practices can circumvent the problems.

These approaches have been considered in upper gastrointestinal cancer since 2001 (Cancer Services Collaborative / Improvement Partnership 2003). Many units have undertaken small projects, which have allowed modification and improvement at local level. Clinical teams have implemented over 50 improvements in upper gastrointestinal cancer care across England. Approximately 70% of upper gastrointestinal cancer patients in CSC projects are now treated within the target waiting time of 62 days from referral to first definitive treatment. Examples of improvements range from scheduling diagnostic and staging procedures on the same day, to standardised CT staging protocols, to improved access to dietary support with dietary information packs, to patient-held diaries and to electronic proformas for transfer of information between unit and centre.

Larger national initiatives are underway, particularly in those parts of the diagnostic pathway where significant delays occur such as endoscopy and radiology. There have been additional benefits to the patients, with greater involvement in their care and opportunity to comment from their experiences. Most units and centres are now planning treatment in multidisciplinary meetings, which significantly raises the standards of service provision and continued professional development.

These approaches have not been without their critics, whose main concerns have been the relative lack of resource to support new initiatives. Some believe that the CSC changes have produced limited peripheral improvements when the main human and capital resources remain unsupported. However, the process can be defended as it does allow a detailed evaluation of the service to identify where improvements can be made. These improvements are often not unique to the originating institution, and the nature of the CSC is such that examples of good practice can be shared between units thus using the available resource in a more efficient and effective way. It also emphasises the importance of good communication between all involved to ensure the service is patient centred whether in primary-, secondary- or tertiary-care settings. It is to be hoped that, as the improvement principles of the CSC become incorporated into routine practices with the introduction of service improvement leads into all networks and service improvement facilitators into all trusts, the concerns over the larger issues can be addressed.

Conclusions

The initiatives proposed in the National Cancer Plan and Improving Outcomes Guidance have been designed to radically alter the way cancer care is delivered. They are undoubtedly ambitious. They require significant changes in working practices, and as a result have been particularly contentious in upper gastrointestinal cancer. However, peer review assessment of the related standards and approaches to service redesign have been embraced by those responsible for planning the services, particularly at network level. As a result, there is already evidence that clinicians are changing working practices and are involved closely in redesign work. There is also evidence of a more patient-focused service, clearly demonstrating that the changes have improved the quality of the patient journey. However, it remains to be seen whether these qualitative improvements will deliver a quantitative improvement in the outcome for patients with a group of cancers that so far have proven difficult to diagnose at an early stage and thus have been associated with limited opportunities for radical curative therapies.

References

Allum, W. H., Griffin, S. M., Watson A. & Colin-Jones, D. G. (2002). Guidelines for the management of oesophageal and gastric cancer. *Gut* **50** (Suppl. V), V1–V23.

Bachmann, M. O., Alderson, D., Edwards, D., Wotton, S., Bedford, C., Peters, T. J. & Harvey, I. M. (2002). Cohort study in South and West England of the influence of specialization on the management and outcome of patients with oesophageal and gastric cancers. *British Journal of Surgery* **89**, 914–922.

Bramhall, S. R., Allum, W. H., Jones, A. G., Allwood, A., Cummins, C. & Neoptolemos, J. P. (1995). Treatment and survival in 13,560 patients with pancreatic cancer, and incidence of the disease in the West Midlands: an epidemiological study. *British Journal of Surgery* **82**, 111–115.

Cancer Services Collaborative / Improvement Partnership (2003). Phase II Progress Report: Upper Gastrointestinal Cancer. NHS Modernisation Agency.

Department of Health (2000). The NHS Cancer Plan – a plan for investment, a plan for reform. London: Department of Health.

Department of Health (2001). Guidance on Commissioning Cancer Services: improving Outcomes in Upper Gastrointestinal Cancers. London: Department of Health.

Department of Health and the Welsh Office (1995). A policy framework for commissioning cancer services. A report by the expert advisory group on cancer to the chief medical officers of England and Wales. Department of Health and the Welsh Office. London: Department of Health.

Fielding, J. W. L., Powell, J., Allum, W. H., Waterhouse, J. A. H. & McConkey, C. C. (eds) (1989). *Clinical Cancer Monographs*, volume 3 (*Cancer of the Stomach*). London: MacMillan.

Hallissey, M. T., Allum, W. H., Jewkes, A. J. *et al.* (1990). Early detection of gastric cancer. *British Medical Journal* **301**, 513–515.

Matthews, H. R., Waterhouse, J. A. H., Powell, J., McConkey, C. C. & Robertson, J. E. (eds) (1987). *Clinical Cancer Monographs*, volume 1 (*Cancer of the Oesophagus*). London: MacMillan.

Neoptolemos, J. P., Russell, R. C. G., Bramhall, S. & Theis, B. for the UK Pancreatic Cancer Group (1997). Low mortality following resection for pancreatic and periampullary tumours in 1026 patients: UK survey of specialist pancreatic units. *British Journal of Surgery* **84**, 1370–1376.

Office for National Statistics (1999). *Mortality Statistics; Cause*. London: Office for National Statistics.

Sue-Ling, H. M., Johnson, D., Martin, I. G. *et al.* (1993). Gastric cancer: a curable disease in Britain. *British Medical Journal* **307**, 591–596.

Index